The Doctor's Communication Handbook

Fifth Edition

Peter Tate

Retired Convenor,
MRCGP Examination

Radcliffe Publishing
Oxford • Seattle

Radcliffe Publishing Ltd
18 Marcham Road
Abingdon
Oxon OX14 1AA
United Kingdom

www.radcliffe-oxford.com
Electronic catalogue and worldwide online ordering facility.

First Edition 1994
Second Edition 1997
Third Edition 2001
Fourth Edition 2003

British Library Cataloguing in Publication Data

A catalogue record for this book is available from the British Library.

ISBN-10: 1 84619 138 6
ISBN-13: 978 1 84619 138 1

Typeset by Anne Joshua & Associates, Oxford
Printed and bound by TJ International Ltd, Padstow, Cornwall

Contents

Preface

When I wrote the first edition of this book in 1994, the intention was to give the reader an easy, up-to-date guide to good communication with patients. There was an ulterior motive, which was to help young GPs taking the then embryonic video examination to understand the criteria and improve their communication skills. Well, both videotape and the examination have nearly run their course in the 12 years that have elapsed since then, and communication has improved, although I confess to being worried about the bad medicine that is sometimes being palmed off with the improved communication skills. Between the fourth edition and this one I have survived serious illness and have been treated wonderfully well by a small army of dedicated NHS staff, the vast majority of whom communicated extremely well. It is to them and their successors in the NHS that this book is dedicated.

This new edition should be especially useful for trainee GPs during the work-based assessment (WBA) part of the nMRCGP, and it will help in the preparation for the Clinical Skills Examination (CSA). It is as up to date as I can make it, and I hope that it will be of use to all doctors in the training part of their careers.

Peter Tate
Retired Convenor, MRCGP Examination
spudtate@supanet.com
September 2006

About the author

Peter Tate qualified at the University of Newcastle in 1968. After spells as a P&O Surgeon and as a trainee in Kentish Town, he worked as a GP in Abingdon for 30 years. He was a trainer from 1976 until 2003, and was also a course organiser in Oxford for eight years. He was an MRCGP examiner from 1981, and was responsible for the introduction of the video module in 1996. He retired as Convenor of the Panel of Examiners in March 2006. He was a co-author of *The Consultation* and *The New Consultation* (both published by Oxford University Press), and has lectured widely on communication issues. He is now semi-retired and lives in Corfe Castle.

Chapter 1

Some early truths to remember

- The patient is as frightened as you are.
- The patient thinks it is more serious than you do.
- Illness is frightening, but understanding what is going on helps. This applies both to the patient and to you.
- Taking a history is a method of controlling what the patient says.

This book is a guide to help you talk with, understand and share with your patients. It will not teach you the traditional medical history-taking model, but it may help you to use that model more effectively both for yourself and for your patients.

Those first encounters with real people who have come to the hospital or the outpatients department for help are very daunting. We all suffer the anxiety of being found wanting, of getting it wrong, of being harshly criticised by our teachers or, worst of all, just looking foolish. *The best way to start is to think ourselves into the role of patient.* After all, this is not too difficult – we have all been ill at some time and we all shall be again. When people become ill they ask themselves several questions, such as 'What has happened?', 'Why has it happened?', 'Why has it happened to me?', 'Why now?', 'What should I do about it?', 'Should I go to the doctor?', 'Is it serious?' and 'Can it be treated?' Think of the last patient you saw. What questions do you think they had asked themselves? Imagine that that patient was you. What would you be asking yourself?

Let us suppose that the last patient you saw was in surgical outpatients and she was a 35-year-old woman presenting to the clinic with a nodular goitre. You have taken her history and found out that she is married with no children. She first noticed a swelling in her neck about six months ago, she went to her GP three months ago, and she has waited for the outpatient appointment since her second visit to the GP two and a half months ago. The GP has stated in his letter that the thyroid function tests were borderline normal and that there is no family history of thyroid disease. In your detailed and systematic history taking you have not discovered any symptoms referable to the thyroid gland, but the patient does seem to be rather anxious. Examination confirms a moderately enlarged gland with multiple small nodules, everything else is normal, but the patient seems to be slightly trembly and perhaps sweating more than you would expect. Now step aside from your history and examination and ask yourself what she might be thinking and feeling. Now do it again.

Let us just consider some of her possible thoughts and feelings. First, she is almost certainly frightened. Hospitals are terrifying places to most people – they are pain and death boxes with a funny smell. She is also afraid of the staff, especially the doctors, *including you*. Doctors are frightening for several reasons, not least their association with the mysteries of life and death. They also tend to be dominant, powerful figures who have control over one's immediate and even long-term future. This patient knows that many doctors do not say very much, and what they do say can be difficult to understand. She also knows that doctors usually do not tell the whole truth.

She is also very concerned about herself. She has a lumpy enlargement in her neck, which to her is cancer until proved otherwise, and she will take a lot of convincing because her aunt died of cancer of the gullet and she had lumps in her neck. She remembers that her aunt's doctors lied to her aunt, and that the treatment was horrible and ineffective. She has heard vaguely about the thyroid gland and knows from a friend that one of the treatments is radioactive. This concerns her because she desperately wants children, she knows time is passing and she fears that a dose of radioactivity may put paid to her chances for ever. She is also afraid of having an operation because she has never been in hospital and hates the idea of being 'put to sleep.' She does not wish to lose control. She also knows from friends, television and everyday experiences that operations go wrong and the neck seems to be a pretty dodgy place. Her husband produced a bundle of printouts from three websites he had found on the Internet about the thyroid gland. She did not understand much of this information, and could not bring herself to read some of the more alarming bits. She wishes that her husband was with her, but worries that he has not really wanted to talk about her neck or her coming to the hospital. She wonders if she is now ugly and unattractive. The bottom line is that she does not want to die.

The above description is only an imaginative guess at some of this patient's feelings, but how much of this did your history reveal, do you think? Is it important to know?

You recite the findings of your history and examination to your chief. She listens and asks both you and your patient (let us call her Mrs Arthur) a few clarifying questions, and examines the thyroid gland herself. She excuses herself to Mrs Arthur and discusses the options with you while the patient listens.

'Multinodular goitre is a difficult clinical area. Probably the best treatment is nothing if the patient can accept the cosmetic deformity. Some centres use thyroxine replacement, but you only get regression in 10–20% of cases. The real patient worry is cancer, isn't that so, Mrs Arthur?' Mrs Arthur, a little startled, nods in agreement. 'Cancer isn't really a problem. The Framingham Study didn't find any in a 15-year follow-up of this sort of goitre, but it remains a theoretical risk, and if you give enough of any thyroid gland to a pathologist he will find some sort of cancer. The real problem we have here with Mrs Arthur is of possible toxicity and the best treatment. The GP's thyroid function tests were borderline high, and Mrs Arthur's clinical state is possibly a little suggestive of hyperactivity. We should repeat the tests and if they are highish give her treatment with radioactive iodine. If that is not successful the next step would be an operation.' She smiles at Mrs Arthur and leaves the room, saying 'The student will explain it all to you. Don't worry, you are in good hands.'

How do you think this patient would cope? What do you think her feelings would be on the way home? What might she say to her husband? Would she come back for the ^{131}I treatment? How helpful was your history? Mrs Arthur will appear again later on, so keep her in mind.

Now think about yourself being unwell again. Imagine waking with a severe sore throat, a lot of swollen neck glands and feeling pretty ropey. Would you go to your GP? If not, what else might make you go? What questions would you ask yourself?

Let us go through some of your possible questions and answers.

1 *What has happened?* It's probably just a virus – Max had it last week.
2 *Why has it happened?* I've been working late, a bit overtired, resistance a bit low.
3 *Why has it happened to me?* Rotten luck, but I always get these things – Max sneezed over me.
4 *What should I do about it?* Dose myself up with soluble aspirin and it should just go.
5 *Is it serious?* No, it will be gone in a few days.

But what happens if the exams are two weeks away or there is a hockey trip to Lanzarote next week?

1 *What has happened?* Maybe it is a streptococcus.
2 *What should I do about it?* I'd better see the GP for some penicillin.
3 *Is it serious?* Yes, if I fail the exam or if I can't make it to Lanzarote.

Or imagine that your partner has glandular fever.

1 *What has happened?* Oh God, it's glandular fever.
2 *Why has it happened?* Too much kissing.
3 *Why has it happened to me?* I had it coming, life has been too good recently.
4 *What should I do about it?* I'd better see the Doc to do a monospot to confirm it.
5 *Is it serious?* Yes, this could put me out for the rest of the year. I've also read that it can cause Hodgkin's disease – oh my God!

These questions and answers can be translated into the trinity of *ideas, concerns* and *expectations*. To continue with the sore throat and glands scenario, consider what *ideas* might be going through your head that first morning:

I feel awful, really really bad, too bad for a cold, it must be at the very least flu. I bet I got it from Max. He was coughing and sneezing all over me last week. It might be streptococcal, so a trip to the GP for some penicillin might help. I wonder if there is any on the ward I could have. I will have to get some soluble aspirin.

What *concerns* might be running through your mind?

Help, I hope and pray it's not glandular fever. If it is, that's the exams down the tubes, and it can lead to Hodgkin's, can't it? What if it's worse? I mean acute leukaemia can start like this. I have been worrying about my immune system for some time. I haven't caught AIDS in casualty, have I? Don't be silly, but it could turn into quinsy like that poor bloke on the ENT ward last week. His tonsils were so big he couldn't breathe. If I don't get this fixed pretty quickly, next week's trip to Lanzarote with the hockey team is finito.

What about your *expectations*?

If I do nothing it will probably go away if I dose myself up, but penicillin is a good idea because it might speed things up, especially with the hockey trip coming up. I expect the old GP will just tell me it's a virus and I will have to lay it on a bit thick to get the penicillin. He might do a blood test for glandular fever. Shall I tell him I'm a bit worried about AIDS? No, he will think I'm being silly. I expect he will tell me off for smoking, too.

Now think about Mrs Arthur again, and consider what sorts of things were going through her mind before she went to her GP for the first time. What she did *not* do was go to him with a nodular goitre. She went because she had certain ideas about the lumpy swelling in her neck. She had several concerns and a few hazy expectations.

*Nobody goes to a doctor with just a symptom. They go with **ideas** about the symptom, with **concerns** about the symptom and with **expectations** related to the symptom.*

Chapter 2

How doctors talk to patients and why

- Asking questions only gets you answers.
- It is not whether the communication between doctor and patient is good or bad that matters, it is whether it is more or less effective.

For over 3000 years now the basic style of doctoring can be described in the modern ethical jargon as beneficent paternalism. The medical profession has thus adopted a well-meaning parental role in most patient encounters. Doctors have acted on behalf of, and for the good of, their patients. They have also wielded power over them. This role, which is taken for granted by our society, produces recognisable patterns of behaviour, which are disease-orientated with a strong tendency towards authoritarianism. It has become clear in recent years that this behaviour affords the doctor some emotional protection – in fact often more perceived than real – and is one of the most important reasons why many doctors find a more sharing approach so difficult.

There has been a great deal of research into doctors' behaviours, and the suggested reading list at the end of this book will help you to explore this area in more detail if you wish to do so.

Agendas

One way to think about the ways in which doctors communicate is to consider the *agendas* for both doctor and patient. Figure 2.1 demonstrates diagrammatically the possible spectrum of doctor communication behaviour with patients.

The right-hand side of the graph is nearly all doctor's agenda, with only the presenting complaint coming from the patient. As the doctor's style moves to the left, more and more of the patient's agenda is taken on board, until at the left-hand end of the graph it is nearly all patient's agenda. Most hospital doctors and still the majority of GPs tend towards the right-hand end of this model. This is not too surprising, as it is the way we are taught. The whole act of *taking* a history is doctor-centred, and not necessarily bad in itself. Medical thoroughness and good pattern recognition are a hallmark of this style when practised well.

As an example of doctor-centred behaviour, imagine Mrs Arthur's first outpatient appointment. It could go something like this:

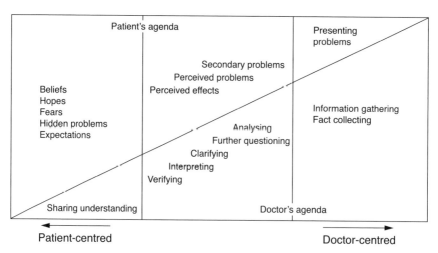

Figure 2.1 A power-shift model of styles of consultation.

> Dr: Good morning, Mrs Arthur. Your GP says you seem to have a problem with your thyroid gland. Tell me, have you lost weight?
>
> Mrs A: No.
>
> Dr: Any hot flushes?
>
> Mrs A: No.
>
> Dr: Feeling tired or slowed up?
>
> Mrs A: Er, well maybe a little, doctor.
>
> Dr: Bowels OK? Not constipated are you?
>
> Mrs A: Not really, doctor, I was wondering . . .
>
> Dr: I think I should examine you now. Would you take your blouse off . . .?

Mrs Arthur's agenda has not figured in the conversation so far – only the doctor's agenda is being addressed.

Here is an example of a more patient-centred style, using the same scenario.

> Dr: Good morning, Mrs Arthur, your GP says you have a problem with your thyroid gland. Would you tell me about it?
>
> Mrs A: Oh, er well yes, I first noticed the swelling a few months ago, but I didn't do anything about it for a while.
>
> Dr: Why not?
>
> Mrs A: Oh, you know, I hoped it would go away while fearing the worst.
>
> Dr: The worst?
>
> Mrs A: Cancer, what else.
>
> Dr: That's a frightening thought. Do you still think it may be cancer?
>
> Mrs A: Well, yes, but I'm hoping you will be able to tell me, doctor.

In this example the patient's agenda figures highly to start with, and the doctor has not yet started on his agenda.

The totally patient-centred doctor is probably a dangerous creature. Patients do after all come for medical advice and considered professional opinions. They don't expect the doctor to let them do all the talking, planning and managing.

However, the first chapter may have got you thinking that the doctor should more often than not take on board some of the patient's belief systems. An ideal doctor might perhaps lie about the middle of this spectrum, changing their behaviour one way or the other depending on the needs of the patient and the situation.

The problem as shown by experience and research work is that doctors *do not change*. Audio and visual recordings of multiple consultations by the same doctor show a remarkable consistency of style. A simple analogy likens us to the traditional Englishman abroad. We don't act differently – we just talk more loudly or slowly. Thus doctors say and do things in much the same way with an anxious 16-year-old coming for a termination as with a 50-year-old woman with menorrhagia or an 80-year-old woman with vulval carcinoma. It appears that we do not regularly adapt to meet the needs of the patient. You could say that this does not matter as long as we have an effective set of behaviours with which we can cope with most patients. However, Chapter 3 will demonstrate that different patients need different types of communication. We need to be flexible, and it appears that most us of are not.

The most basic communication need is to discover why our patient has come to see us. This seems almost too obvious to state, but much research work suggests that doctors are not very good at it. In many consultations, doctors and patients do not appear to be talking about the same thing. Many years ago one of the truly great academic GPs, Professor Pat Byrne, gave this type of consultation the deliberately ugly name of *dysfunctional*. In this sort of consultation the doctor and the patient are pursuing their own quite separate agendas.

Doctors are good at diagnosis (i.e. establishing in the medical sense why a patient has come to see them). We discover the nature and history of the problem and the likely cause, but we tend not to be good at searching out our patients' beliefs and expectations. These are the real reasons why patients come to see us, and not discovering them can lead to a mismatch of agendas.

For example, a gloomy 64-year-old man comes to his GP for a sick note. The doctor knows this patient to be a somewhat aggressive, paranoid depressive with a long history of repeated admissions to a psychiatric hospital. The man says that he has been in hospital recently and asks for a certificate. The doctor, seeing no record of the latest admission, but assuming that the usual has occurred, acquiesces quickly. He wants to avoid any difficult confrontation, and therefore signs a certificate stating 'depression.' The doctor and patient briefly discuss convalescence and returning to work, and the patient leaves.

What is wrong with this scenario? Almost everything! The whole consultation was based on a false premise. The patient had in fact been admitted to hospital with a myocardial infarction. The doctor's original assumption was false, and nothing in the ensuing communication put it right. The doctor had failed to discover why his patient was there, and the patient did not realise this.

Dysfunctional consultations are common in general practice because the patient's reason for coming to see their doctor is often unclear, but major misunderstandings do occur regularly in hospital. Consider the case of Mrs Arthur again. Let us carry on with the doctor-centred example given earlier in this chapter. Assume that the doctor has examined Mrs Arthur and completed the history taking in the form of a series of staccato questions. Mrs Arthur has therefore contributed none of her own thoughts and feelings. The time for explanation and management has come.

> Dr: Well, Mrs Arthur, there is nothing to worry about. You have multinodular goitre, but this is a benign condition. There are a couple more tests we need to do just to be on the safe side. I will arrange for a special scan and a biopsy of that biggish lump. Is that OK?
>
> Mrs A: So you are sure it is not serious, doctor?
>
> Dr: Oh yes. Speak to the nurse about the arrangements for the tests and I will see you in a month. Goodbye.
>
> Mrs A: Well, goodbye doctor, er thank you.

This is deficient communication. The patient has not had any of her agenda addressed. Consider her ideas in Chapter 1. She has not been reassured about her future. She will probably attend for the tests out of fear, but she may default. She is not sure what the words 'multi-nodular', 'goitre', 'benign', 'special scan' or 'biopsy' mean, and she will go home feeling frustrated and afraid. The doctor, in turn, has focused his attention on the thyroid gland to the exclusion of everything else. He knows little about Mrs Arthur and nothing about her specific fears or reasons for consulting. This consultation is truly dysfunctional.

Power

Look at Figure 2.1 again and think about *power*. This type of diagram is known as a power-shift model. The doctor is much more in control on the right-hand side, and his power slips away as the agenda increasingly becomes that of the patient. This is not to say that the totally patient-centred doctor does not have power. They simply have less direct control and are much less authoritarian. It is worth stopping here to consider the nature of doctor power.

Patients expect and often want a powerful doctor – that is, a doctor who has reassuring authority, who is apparently capable and whose pronouncements can reduce anxiety. One definition of medical or 'Aesculapean' authority divides it into three parts – *sapiental, moral* and *charismatic*. These words are somewhat offputting at first meeting, but bear with me.

Sapiental authority

This can be defined as the right to be heard, based on knowledge or expertise, and it means that doctors must know, or at least appear to know, more about medicine than their patients. However, this can only be one part of the doctor's authority, as a biochemist may know more about a particular branch of medicine, but it is to a physician that a patient turns when they are in need.

Moral authority

This is the right to control and direct patients significantly, based on doing what society expects of us as doctors. In order to retain their moral authority, doctors must always act with the good of the patient as their paramount concern. This is derived from the Hippocratic credo. In addition, societies generally revere doctors – that is, their behaviour is seen as socially right as well as individually good. This is a powerful combination.

Charismatic authority

This is the most difficult of the three concepts, and is similar to the anthropological definition of magic. It stems from the original unity between medicine and religion. In Western culture it is related to the possibility of death, and the magnitude of the issues with which the doctor deals. Many patients want doctors to be a little magical. For many patients there is a need to supplement sapiental and moral authority with an ineffable factor, which might just hold out hope against the odds. Many doctors go out of their way to cultivate this. They develop a priestly mien, use complicated and obscure rituals, and act more like bishops than physicians.

The three forms of authority are present in all doctors, although some doctors go out of their way to develop particular sapiental, moral and charismatic elements in their behaviour with patients and others. Think about some of the powerful doctors you have met and the nature of their power.

Here is an example. A partially patient-centred doctor, like that shown in Figure 2.1, has the same moral authority as their doctor-centred colleague, but they may reduce some of their sapiental authority by sharing more information with their patients. This highlights a fundamental truth. *Controlling information increases doctor power and restricts patient involvement.* Many doctors become very uneasy with knowledgeable and inquisitive patients, as such patients decrease the doctor's control. The partially patient-centred doctor will also be more likely to attempt to demystify the nature of medical diagnosis and treatment, reducing their charismatic authority and thus their power to control the interview. This requires a degree of bravery, particularly when first trying such strategies.

Many doctors, perhaps especially when they are training, are afraid of losing control – of exposing too much of their patient's pain and fear. You may find yourself not asking the important question due to fear of opening an emotional Pandora's box and becoming overwhelmed. Such doctors use their power over their patient to keep the box shut and emotions at a non-threatening level. This style of behaviour can then become fixed and persist throughout a career. Don't let this happen to you, or you will lose much more than you will gain.

Doctors can increase their charismatic power, should they wish to do so, in many different ways. The trappings of power are the most obvious – for example, white coats, impressive mysterious gadgetry, attached (subservient) staff, a large desk with a big chair placed firmly behind it, grandiose-looking certificates on the wall, and computers with unintelligible displays or pointing away from the patient. They may communicate by means of cryptic oracle-like pronouncements, shrouded in 'medico-speak.' This can then be wrapped up with dire warnings of the fearsome consequences of not following the treatment properly, in order to complete the effect. Powerful rituals such as examining and prescribing are more charismatic in the absence of adequate explanations.

The problem with this contrived exercise of medical authority is that the overwhelming evidence suggests that *it is not very effective*. It quite obviously does not increase patient understanding, because that is not what is motivating the doctor. The often-quoted reason for this style of communication is that it will make patients do what is good for them. However, the sad fact of the matter is that more often than not they don't. The literature on compliance or what is now more hopefully called *concordance* with medical advice reflects rather badly on doctors.

The *rule of one-thirds* describes this. It is easy to remember and is well authenticated.

- One-third of patients take medical advice and act in accordance with it sufficient for the advice to be effective.
- One-third take heed of some of the advice, but not enough for it to be effective. Imagine the way that many doctors take pills for a sore

throat – a few one day when it is sore, forget for a day a day or so, and then start again when the throat gets sore again.
- One-third just don't bother.

For the fifth edition of this handbook it would be encouraging to report that recent evidence has shown this trend to be improving. Sadly this is still not so. In many cases the rule of thirds appears to err greatly on the optimistic side.

Take the common life-threatening condition of maturity-onset diabetes, an illness that leads to blindness, terrible circulatory problems and considerable morbidity. Many patients need at least two drugs to control their blood-sugar level adequately. The modern rash of protocols usually assumes 100% adherence to prescribing regimes. So what are the facts? In a careful and thorough study of 1000 diabetic patients from Tayside in Scotland, reported in early 2000, the authors showed that adherence to a one-drug regime did indeed fit the rule of thirds, with 33% of patients taking the medication as prescribed. However, when two drugs were prescribed the adherence rate fell to 13%! A review of the literature in 2005 revealed that long-term adherence to drug treatment decreased over time, and that 50% was an average figure after 3 years.

Think about this long and hard. You want to be the finest doctor in the land – to be able to recognise a yellow nail syndrome at 20 feet, to restore ailing people to full vigour with your hard-earned expertise – but in some cases more than two-thirds of your patients don't follow your advice. If your patients are really like that, how much use are you? How can you make sure that this fate won't befall you? Do you have to be in absolute control?

There is now a healthy debate about the very word 'compliance', which implies a subservient relationship. As previously mentioned, many experts are now advocating the use of the word 'concordance' instead, and some prefer the word 'adherence.' What is clear is that the slavish following of medical advice by patients is not only an unusual behaviour, but appears to be so uncommon in many cases as to be regarded as deviant.

Now think about this. You are living through a time of historic change in the role of doctors. You are no longer the keeper of occult secrets, you are not the fount of all medical wisdom, and many of your patients will know more about their individual disease than you carry in your head. Your job has changed as you are now your patients' medical interpreter. The Internet has torn up the rules, old-fashioned communication strategies are no longer viable, shared decision making is a must, and concordance rules. Read on.

Chapter 3

Different types of patient

- The same words will often mean different things to different people.
- Patients are people, and they are all different.
- What works for one patient probably won't work for another.
- What is most important is what matters to patients.

The health belief model

This is the most researched and validated description of patients' beliefs about health and related matters, and it has five main elements.

1 People's interest in their health and the degree to which they are motivated to change it (*health motivation*) varies enormously.
2 When considering specific health problems, people think very differently about how likely they are to be affected (*perceived vulnerability*). For example, people who think that they are at high risk of developing lung cancer are more likely to follow advice about giving up smoking than those who do not think they are at risk.

   If a patient already has a health problem, then their perceived vulnerability relates to the degree to which they believe in the diagnosis and its possible consequences.

   For example, a patient may be diagnosed in the gastroenterology clinic as having irritable bowel syndrome, and it is suggested that tension may be contributing to the condition. However, if the patient is convinced that pelvic inflammatory disease and not tension is the cause, they are unlikely to adhere to the proposed management plan. This disbelief in what they are told may not be explicit and needs to be searched for. They do not regard themselves as being susceptible to tension, and they therefore conclude that there must be another cause. Most probably they have pelvic inflammatory disease like their friend, they think, and the doctor must be wrong.

3 Patients vary in how dire they believe the consequences of contracting a particular illness or of leaving it untreated (*perceived seriousness*) would be.

Heart disease or lung cancer may seem to be a very remote possibility to a 16-year-old girl who is starting to smoke because of peer pressure. Her attitude may be 'And anyway by the time I get to 40 they will have a cure for it, won't they?'

On the other hand, the publicity about skin cancer resulting from ozone depletion has meant that, in recent years, anxious patients have flocked to doctors with a wide range of minor skin blemishes. I see one such patient in almost every surgery. Most people regard cancer as very serious, and some, if they suspect it, may even be too frightened to go to the doctor. Particularly sad examples of this situation, which unfortunately are not uncommon, include older women with slowly growing fungating carcinomas of the breast. Young men with testicular growths do appear to have benefited from the publicity about testicular cancer, and now seem more likely to attend than was previously the case.

4 Patients weigh up the advantages and disadvantages of taking any particular course of action, not necessarily taking all of the relevant considerations into account, but making an evaluation nonetheless (*perceived costs and benefits*). This cost–benefit analysis is unique to each individual, and can be influenced by outsiders, including doctors. However, in order to influence the equation in the patient's favour, those factors that are already included by the patient need to be known by the doctor. Consider Mrs Arthur and the possibility of ^{131}I treatment. Her fear that radiation would prevent her from conceiving might stop her complying with the treatment because in her own mind the risks of

treatment outweigh the benefits. Thus it becomes imperative for the doctor to seek out such fears and talk them through with her.

5   Patients' beliefs do not already exist in a pre-packaged form. They are prompted or created by a number of stimuli and triggers (*cues to action*), such as a physical sensation, what Granny said, a television programme or what has just happened to the man down the road.

The health belief model emphasises what we have already discussed. People are generally engaged in a struggle to understand what is happening to them as well as what might happen. Different people try to resolve these dilemmas in different ways. Each person's belief system is of course unique, but it is strongly influenced by race, culture, religion and the immediate society. A poor Chinese peasant will have a very different health understanding to a German banker, but so will people living in the same environment. There will be little similarity between the health understanding of a Geordie miner and a black Rastafarian, both living in Newcastle. There are major differences between peoples in different strata of the same society, and the differences are often still considerable within the same social group.

The health belief model threw up another concept, namely *locus of control*. This is jargon for how we explain to ourselves what is likely to happen to our health. Using this idea we can divide the human race into three types of people. Each of these will now be described in turn.

The internal controller

This type of person believes that fundamentally they are in charge of their own future health. In other words, what happens to their health is largely the result of their own actions. This is the muesli-eating, brown rice and leather sandal brigade – those diligent humans who digest every morsel of health-related news from the *Guardian* or *Telegraph* health page. They will not have an aluminium pot in the house for fear of Alzheimer's disease, and are to be found sweating in health-food shops, rummaging for the elixir of life, having just jogged five miles to get there. There are certain implications for this type of believer, not least that they tend to get very cross if they do get ill. To spend 20 years abstaining from the good things in life in order to keep one's cholesterol level below 5 mmol/litre and then still have a coronary at the age of 55 results in a very unhappy and disillusioned human being.

As far as communication is concerned, this type of person likes explanations, dialogue and Socratic discourse. They want to be involved in decisions about their health and they want to know what is happening. The medical arguments and explanations do not necessarily need to be rational. This group is enthusiastic about alternative medicine and, let's face it, a great many medical explanations are at best dubious and sometimes downright wrong, but if they are convincing the internal controller will accept them.

The external controller

This type of person is the opposite of the internal controller. They do not believe that they have any control over their health. What will be will be. They are fatalists. A good example is the 'bullet with my name on' type of person who can be found down at the local pub expounding their theories as to why these dietary, high exercise, low fat and no alcohol theories much loved by the medical profession are rubbish.

> My grandfather lived to be 95 and he smoked 10 large King Edward cigars a day, washed down with a bottle of Martell, he had clotted cream with everything and was shot in bed with his 25-year-old mistress by her jealous husband, etc.

In my career the most explicit external controller I have ever met was a fortyish, unfit mechanic with an expanding paunch who was complaining of feeling rather run down. Among other things I gently enquired about exercise and his proclivity towards it. He knew immediately what I was trying to say:

> You're not talking about jogging are you, Doc? I'm not for that at all. Look, I reckon in this life God gives you a certain number of heartbeats and I'm buggered if I'm wasting any of mine running round in bloody circles on wet Sunday mornings!

An external controller is not keen on Socratic dialogue, or at least not as far as their health is concerned. They want to be told what to do and then to ignore the advice or not as the case may be. They are not really much into involvement, and take little or no interest in the media obsession with health matters. Curiously, research in this field suggests that people with an external locus of control are more likely to be influenced by the simplistic vast poster campaigns, much practised by well-intentioned but misguided organisations such as the now defunct Health Education Council, exhorting people to avoid a variety of pleasurable but possibly dangerous activities.

It is most important for us to remember that the form of communication which will work best with the internal controller will not work well with the external controller. Now we come to the third type of person.

The powerful other

This type is quite different from the other two. They do not believe that they are in control of their own health, nor are they fatalists. They believe that *you* are in charge of their health.

> I have this terrible cough, doctor. I know it's not related to my smoking because I have been doing that for a long time and it has never bothered me. I'd like you to give me something to stop it.

Doctors, of course, see a disproportionate number of this type of person. Many of those individuals that have been described as 'heartsink' patients can be found in this category.

The powerful others of this world pose another difficult challenge for us doctors. Strategies that involve trying to give such patients more responsibility for their own health are firmly resisted. Getting them involved in deciding how to proceed is also difficult, as powerful others are quite firm about their agenda for the doctor, and are at their happiest with authoritarian doctors who relieve them of any responsibility for their own health. They are not easily educated, and if their agenda for their health does not coincide with that of the doctor, they will not follow the medical advice that they are given.

Some examples of patients with different loci

Mrs Cheshire is a 50-year-old, 19-stone smoker who hates doctors.

> Mrs Cheshire: I've come about my knees, doctor. Something's got to be done, I can't go on like this.
> Dr: [with an outward sigh and an inner scream] Mrs Cheshire, you know the problem, you really must lose weight. I can't do anything for those knees till you have at least two stone off. I am sending you to the dietitian and then I want regular weighing by our nurse to keep you on the straight and narrow.

Why doesn't this work? Mrs Cheshire wants relief from pain, a touch of medicinal magic, something fairly easy. She is well aware of her lifelong weight problem, does not think it is that relevant, and certainly does not want the usual doctor response she has heard since her twenties. She thinks that it is her doctor's responsibility to cure her pain, not hers. Unfortunately you, her doctor, disagree on nearly all counts. Your agendas are mismatched and you think that Mrs Cheshire should take responsibility for her illness – that she can, should and will lose weight, and as a result her knees will improve.

You think that the illness is her own fault. This will remain a difficult consultation or series of consultations until one of you is prepared to change agendas. Can you do it? Should you? This woman believes that her health is your responsibility. She is a 'powerful other.'

Here is another common example of a powerful other locus. Miss Moore is a 25-year-old, chronically nervous individual with a set of notes already larger than average, mainly full of minor illness and over-investigated vague complaints. A shortened version of your conversation is as follows.

> Miss Moore: Doctor, I am very worried. I am tired all the time and my boyfriend says there must be something seriously wrong with me. Do you think it is my virus again?
> Dr: [wearily, and with a resigned but worldly-wise air] No, it's not your virus. We have talked about this before – you worry too much. Stop worrying about yourself and go out and enjoy yourself. There is nothing wrong with you.

You are almost certainly right, but you see her the next evening coming out of your partner's surgery. Why? Perhaps because she wanted you to take on board her fears, take on responsibility for her unwellness and give her a nice neat little physical illness with a label to wave at her boyfriend. You did not want to do any of this. What else might you have done? You had made a good start by recognising her agenda and then overruling it with good reason. Perhaps this was too much of a one-way process. You could recognise her agenda, but she either did not accept or did not wish to be a part of your agenda. There was no negotiation, no 'give and take', no sweetening of the message. A little intelligent sympathy thrown in might help. For example:

> It's rotten feeling tired all the time, everything's an effort. Tell me how it affects you . . . you must find it worrying feeling like this . . . what do you think might be going on? . . . I often find when someone tells me they are feeling like you do that really they are feeling a bit down and miserable. Are you?

How do you cope with another common and difficult consultation? Here we have introspective, fussy Mr Fogarty with a list of minor ailments and a host of strategies for dealing with them, all of which he wants to discuss.

> Do you think I should be taking zinc tablets for my heart? Remember my cholesterol last month was 5.6. Can you remeasure it to see if my walnut and avocado diet is really working?

This man's agenda clearly relates to him being in control of his health – a definite internal controller, but with a desire for a lot of your involvement and a distinct whiff of hypochondria. What is your agenda? Is it to get him out of the room as fast as possible, to help him to educate himself, or to train him to use your services in a reasonable way?

Let us think about your agenda again. Perhaps you are a well-meaning intervening preventionist, using every opportunity you can to attack obesity, smoking and sloth. Mr Reid, an external controller par excellence, comes to you with a sore throat, smelling of old beer and cigarettes, and knocks over your sphygmomanometer with his swinging gut.

> Come on, doc, out with the penicillin and none of your lectures.

What now? There are myriads of strategies you could try, depending on your inner agenda, but which of them will work? What will satisfy you and yet help your patient?

Influencing locus of control

When Mrs Arthur first went to her GP she had prepared her speech, but she did not feel in control of the situation, nor was she fatalistic. She wanted the doctor to take the lead, but she did expect a referral and an explanation. She could not be pigeon-holed into any of the three categories described above, but perhaps is closest to a powerful other who, with support, judicious involvement and some education, can be helped to take more control over her worrying illness.

The good thing about locus of control as far as doctors are concerned is that it can be influenced. It is rather like political affiliation – most of us lean to the left or the right, but can sometimes be cajoled to vote the other way. Similarly, locus of control in most people is a tendency, not a fixed aspect of their personality. A further point about external or internal beliefs about health matters is that we humans are not necessarily consistent. For example, I may be at heart more or less a fatalist, but I still buy big chunky cars, believing them to be safer for my family and perhaps for me.

If it is correct that the communication strategy of the medical profession should be directed towards increasing people's tendency to look after their own health and take some responsibility for their health – and I believe that it should – only the internal controllers are going to accept this idea readily. The other 50–60% of patients are going to need some persuading. However, the effort may be worthwhile for several reasons, not least because it is likely to lead to more patients following more medical advice. In a review of the literature in 2001 it was found that for five behaviours, the odds of healthy behaviour were more than 40% higher among individuals in the internal controller category. Fatalist scores were associated with a reduction of more than 20% in the likelihood of healthy options for six behaviours, while powerful others' scores showed more variable associations with healthy actions.

Now a cautionary thought about control. Consider type 1 diabetes. Many young female diabetics quickly discover that letting their sugar levels rise produces weight loss – high sugar equals small bum. So they make a conscious risk decision to put their health at risk in the long term in order to obtain a short-term reward. Is this internal control or fatalism? It is certainly common – ask your diabetic patients.

If patients all require different styles of communication depending on their locus of control, and research suggests that we doctors have on balance pretty inflexible styles; then how are we, as doctors, going to acquire the necessary flexibility without spending all our lives at communication workshops? Heaven forbid.

The answer must be to explore our patients' agendas. If we know their beliefs, and have an inkling about their locus of control, we can try to follow at least some, if not necessarily all, of their agenda, and talk to them about what matters to them and to us. Communication will therefore become tailored to the individual and will thus automatically become more flexible.

During the interval between the publication of the fourth and fifth editions of this book I was very ill for a while, and in Appendix 2 you will find my own slightly wry take on how it went for me. However, I shall close this chapter with a quote from another doctor who wrote about his own illness in the *British Medical Journal*.

- The information that I want is not that 1 in 10 patients will benefit, but whether I am that one.
- When I return to practice after my treatment, I shall ensure that I focus on the individual in front of me and my traditional consulting skills.

Shelford G. Personal view. *BMJ.* 2003; **327**: 757.

Chapter 4

The patient's learning circle

> The White Rabbit put on his spectacles. 'Where shall I begin please your Majesty?' he asked.
> 'Begin at the beginning,' the King said gravely, 'and go on till you come to the end: then stop.'

David Pendleton first demonstrated this idea to me in 1980, and we used it in the book, *The Consultation: an approach to learning and teaching* (published by Oxford University Press in 1984), and again in *The New Consultation* (published by Oxford University Press in 2003).

When patients meet doctors and some form of communication takes place, they are changed – not necessarily in ways that doctors may hope for or expect, but some change in understanding does occur. It is important for us to analyse the effects that our contacts with our patients have on their subsequent behaviour and beliefs about health and illness (*see* Figure 4.1).

In the previous chapters we have thought about some of the issues that affect patients' decisions to consult, and what factors make up their health understanding. It is now time to consider the role of doctors as educators in this learning circle. Let us start with the outcomes.

Commitment to plan

After a patient has consulted you, they come away with immediate decisions on whether to follow your advice or not. There are many

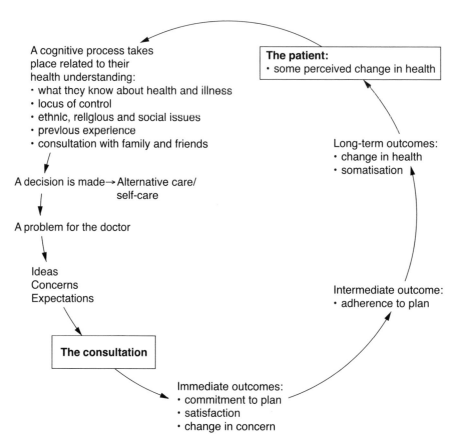

Figure 4.1 The patient's learning circle.

reasons why they may follow your advice. The first and best is that they believe and understand you, and that their agendas approximate closely to yours. Other reasons include doing what one is told by a respected professional. This may result in the idea that it was not quite what they were expecting, but you are the doctor so they will give it a try. Alternatively, they may just be too frightened to disobey.

The problem, as described at the end of Chapter 2, is that 50% or more of patients do not follow our advice closely and are not committed to the plan, most probably because it is our plan and not theirs. Consider the following example.

A 54-year-old man is referred to the cardiology clinic by his GP with a letter saying 'This man has developed intermittent chest pain over the last 3/12 that has some cardiac features, such as being related to exercise and radiating to his left arm. His resting ECG is normal, BP is 150/85, and I can't find anything obviously wrong. He smokes 20 a day and is a line worker at the car plant. There is no past history of anything significant.'

The clinic is rushed as usual, but you take his history in more detail and examine him thoroughly. Like the GP, you think that there may be an element of angina, and you arrange for him to return for a treadmill test and give him some glyceryl trinitrate tablets to take under his tongue when the pain begins. Later you are surprised to hear that he defaulted from the treadmill test. Why did he default?

In this case, the reason was simple. He thought that you and his GP were investigating the wrong thing. He went to his GP with chest pains, worried that they heralded the onset of oesophageal cancer because his father had presented in the same way. The possibility that the pain might be related to his heart had occurred to him, but it did not correspond to his idea of heart pain. He was confused that his GP did not mention cancer or ask him about his throat, but he was worried that his GP really did think it was cancer because he sent him to the hospital. He kept his appointment because he thought that the hospital would do tests that would rule out cancer. When he found out that you at the hospital were like his GP – only interested in his heart – he did not feel committed to your plan. He assumed that you were not worried about cancer. He was not concerned about his heart, so he decided to do nothing unless something else developed, in which case he would go back to his GP.

Take asthma as another example. An article published in the journal *Chest* in 2006 demonstrated that a single question effectively identifies those who don't think their asthma is a chronic disease, and therefore don't manage it as one: 'Do you think you have asthma all the time, or only when you are having symptoms?' In total, 53% of hospital admissions in this study held the 'no symptoms, no asthma' belief.

Change in concern

The immediate thought that most of us have is that going to a doctor will reduce our concern. However, this is often not true of course. Let us take a simple headache as an example.

In the town in which I work, probably 100 people wake up each morning with a headache, and one or two of them come to the doctor. They usually, but not always, turn out to be the most concerned of the 100 individuals.

The first is a 25-year-old woman who is afraid of her recurrent headaches, and thinks that she probably has a brain tumour. She is hoping to be taken seriously and properly investigated and treated. She has come today because the headache is particularly bad, and she had a row with her boyfriend last night over a television programme about doctors misdiagnosing cancers. I am rushed, and although I do not discover all of this, I do discover her fear of a brain tumour and see her immense relief at being allowed to talk about it. I examine her thoroughly, including her fundi. This is, of course, intended to be both diagnostic and therapeutic. After discussion, explanation, advice and the offer of a possible follow-up appointment, she leaves with less concern than when she arrived. Her health understanding has changed a little, but the change is brittle and it will not take much to bring her back.

Our second patient is a 56-year-old banker who says that he is not too concerned about his recent onset of migraines because his mother got them at about this age, but he would like some of those new injections or something like that which he read about in the evening paper. We go through the same routine. This time I notice a nystagmus to the left and papilloedema of the left disc with a fuzzy right disc. He picks up on my concern, and the urgent need for a neurological opinion raises his anxiety level considerably.

This is a rare event in general practice – most headaches are not caused by brain tumours. This example is intended to illustrate the rather obvious point that concern can increase after a successful consultation. This point, although not subtle, needs to be borne in mind when reading learned papers about changes in concern.

Let us now return to Mrs Arthur. When she first went to her GP, he examined her thyroid thoroughly and did a blood test. He did not mention cancer and neither did she. Did he not mention it because he thought it was cancer and didn't want to frighten her? Was the blood test for cancer? He did say something about going to hospital. Was that in order to see a cancer specialist? Mrs Arthur was not less concerned on leaving.

Remember the interchange at the hospital. How do you think Mrs Arthur's concern changed? If she is very concerned about possible ^{131}I treatment, and nothing you have said has alleviated this concern, then her health understanding remains unchanged and she is likely to default.

The effect that the doctor's style can have on the patient's concern is worth repeating. Respected authoritarian physicians have the power to reduce anxiety at the cost of reducing patient autonomy, and this effect is sometimes short-lived. However, giving ill patients too much autonomy can increase their anxiety. This is a difficult equation and it deserves your attention. Sharing information and understanding would seem to be the best compromise, as this approach is most likely to increase autonomy while constraining any increase in concern.

The last point about concern relates to a curve that is well known and much loved by psychologists (*see* Figure 4.2).

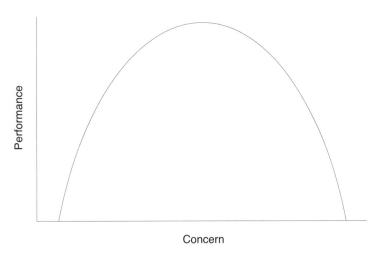

Figure 4.2 Concern measured against performance.

As you can see, performance increases with concern up to a certain point, and then plateaus and falls off. This curve should interest doctors, too. If the anxiety or concern is too great, patients will not do what it is in their best interest to do. This may be why showing rotting cancerous lungs in bottles to smokers is not usually a very effective technique for helping them to give up. It pushes the majority over the top of the curve. Too great a fear of cancer freezes patients into inertia, and usually stops them hearing you, too, whereas a small decrease in concern may put them on peak performance to enable them to face the rigours of the treatment. This is a simple but very important curve. Keep it in mind.

Satisfaction

This is a commonly measured factor in many articles about doctor–patient communication. The simple equation is high satisfaction = good, and low satisfaction = bad. However, as usual, life is not quite that straightforward. Many health messages are not particularly satisfying, even if a jury of peers would concur with them, the continuing craze for lifestyle advice, enhanced in the UK by a payment system reinforcing such doctor behaviour, being an obvious example. The patient comes to her GP with a cough and is told to stop smoking, lose weight, and have her cervix smeared, her breasts examined and her cholesterol level measured, and is then told that she cannot have any cough mixture prescribed. To a large section of the community this may be profoundly unsatisfying, but to the majority of the profession this would now be seen as good practice, and certainly lucrative.

There is an easy way to satisfy most patients, and that is to give them what they want. Most alternative therapies work on this principle. The traditional Baked Bean healing strategy works on the principle of the healer always having an answer and always satisfying the patient.

- My dear, I am glad you are improving. Let's increase the dose of the Baked Beans.

- Don't worry that you have not improved. Let's use the very special sun-dried African Beans hand picked in the Kalahari.
- I'm sure we can help you if we just cut the dose by a tiny amount.

Thus there is either the right dose, too much, too little or the wrong sort. Doctors are not immune from this behaviour, but they tend not to be as good at it.

The fact that patients often want treatments such as unnecessary antibiotics, excessive time, more of you than you can spare, dubious operations, etc., means that the goal of only satisfying patients is a poor one. We need more integrity than that. Again, it becomes obvious that patient satisfaction is a subtle measure and needs to be interpreted carefully.

Some facts about satisfaction are clear. A patient's satisfaction with the consultation is strongly influenced by the amount of information that they are given. A 1998 review of over 40 studies of patient satisfaction showed that information provision by the doctor was positively associated with patient satisfaction, as was patient information giving, although high levels of closed questions seemed to produce more negative results. Unsurprisingly, doctors' friendliness, courtesy and expression of warm and positive feelings in consultations were positively associated with patient satisfaction, whereas the expression of negative feelings (irritation, anger, etc.) was associated with patient dissatisfaction.

In 1997, in a primary care study of 716 consultations involving a sore throat, Little and colleagues demonstrated that patients who were more satisfied got better more quickly, and satisfaction was strongly correlated with how well the doctor dealt with the patient's concerns. They went on to point out that this was not easy.

Thus it seems that satisfying our patients is important because the evidence shows that satisfied patients are more likely to follow medical advice. There is little evidence that time makes much difference, but communication and style do. It seems to be the case that warm, friendly doctors are more likely to satisfy patients than cold, businesslike ones. In the jargon, 'positive affect' works well. It also appears that a doctor talking too much reduces satisfaction, whereas the sense of being listened to and understood increases it. Therefore it is really not difficult – patients like doctors who smile at them, are friendly and actively listen to them, and within this framework will then accept some of the less pleasant health messages without becoming fed up.

Intermediate outcomes: concordance, compliance or adherence

There is a difference between the 'commitment to plan', immediate decisions about adherence and the full follow-through to complete the course. Defaulting can occur at any of these stages. The poor uptake of medical advice remains a major challenge to our profession, but it could be argued that within many patients' health understanding there lurks a healthy scepticism about medical advice, and that if we as doctors really do wish to influence our patients to do what we think is good for them, we had better be very certain that we are right.

The patient is more likely to adhere to treatment if they understand and believe the explanation. Some patients will adhere simply because it is a doctor who has told them to. Most will adhere if their own understanding seems to match that of the doctor and their agenda is shared – this is what is meant by concordance. A shared understanding should be a general professional goal. A whole issue of the *British Medical Journal*, entitled 'From compliance to concordance' (11 October 2003), was devoted to this topic.

There is a fascinating area that we doctors know very little about, namely what lessons our patients learn from whether they follow our advice or not (*see* Table 4.1).

Around 99% of patients act rationally in terms of their own health beliefs which, however, may not themselves be rational. For

Table 4.1 The effect of adherence on understanding

	Patient gets well	*Patient does not get well*
Patient adheres to treatment	A	B
Patient does not adhere to treatment	C	D

example, patient A goes to the doctor wanting penicillin for her sore throat. She is given it, gets better and has her health belief confirmed – that penicillin cures sore throats. Patient B does exactly the same but does not get better. What lessons has he learned? That penicillin does not cure sore throats? That it was not a 'strong' enough antibiotic and that the doctor was ineffective in choosing the right one? For example, 'I've always had the green ones before – these red ones are useless.' That the doctor was right all the time and it was a virus that did not respond to penicillin? That there may be something very serious that the doctor missed? That this doctor is no good and that he will try another one next time? And so on. There is another possibility with patient B, namely partial compliance. He might be one of the third of patients who take a few pills here and there, but not enough to achieve adequate blood levels (but he may still think that he has followed the doctor's instructions).

What about patient C? He only came for a sick note, but was given tablets that he did not want, did not take, and he got better. 'I don't know what they teach doctors at medical school, always giving pills for no good reason.' Or patient D? She was given penicillin but did not take it because it had given her thrush last time, but now she feels both unwell and guilty. If she goes back to the doctor she might well lie about taking the tablets. These are just some examples of the types of message that our patients learn from whether they do or do not take our advice. How many of these types of message are we aware of?

Let us go back to Mrs Arthur and put her in each of these boxes, and assume that she has a borderline toxic goitre.

In Box A, treatment with ^{131}I is agreed upon. Mrs Arthur's fears about infertility are dispelled, and she complies with the treatment, which is unpleasant but she has been prepared for it. She feels a little better and is grateful for your attention. She still worries about the lumps, but is now more likely to accept any further recommendations, such as an operation.

In Box B, she has an unpleasant reaction to the treatment and feels quite poorly. She is totally unprepared, having had little or no explanation of what the treatment entails, and she is horrified that she had to stay in a little side-ward away from anyone else, and that even her husband was only allowed to see her through a leaded hatch. No one really talked to her during the three unpleasant days she spent in the hospital, and her food was taken away by staff wearing masks and rubber gloves. She is now more convinced than ever that she will definitely be infertile, and she wonders whether you have made an incorrect diagnosis or whether your management was wrong. She is not happy with the hospital and may default any further follow-up.

In Box C, Mrs Arthur refuses to come for ^{131}I treatment because of her fears. Anyway, she feels fine now, and she thinks that you ordered a dangerous and unnecessary treatment. She has little faith in your opinion that she does or does not need an operation. She may go back to her GP for their opinion, but the GP is also tarnished in her eyes for sending her to that hospital in the first place.

In Box D, Mrs Arthur refuses to come for ^{131}I treatment for the same reasons as in Box C, but finds herself losing more and more weight. She becomes increasingly frightened but is afraid to call her own GP because she has not followed medical advice.

Of course, the changing pattern of her illness can easily move her from box to box, constantly altering what she is learning from these experiences. Her health understanding will be changed by each meeting with her doctors and by the outcomes of those meetings.

A major problem with communication between doctor and patient concerns the different frames of reference. Doctors are taught scientifically, learn thousands of new words and have models of disease imprinted in their brains. Patients are not like this. Both doctors and patients have reasons for believing and doing what they do – the trouble is that these reasons are different. For example, consider hypertension, a doctor's disease if ever there was one. Until the advent of cheap electronic machines, only professionals could diagnose this condition. Doctors insist to their patients that high blood pressure produces no symptoms and can only be effectively treated by regular medication and frequent monitoring. This is the concept of the asymptomatic risk factor. Most patients cannot understand this approach and use more obvious folk explanations to help them to cope with what they perceive as an illness. The result is the adherence nightmare alluded to earlier. Most patients think that hypertension is a description, and take their medication depending on how they feel. If they are feeling headachy, a bit tense and edgy, then to them it is obvious that they are hypertensive and need to take their tablets, but on days when they are feeling serene and relaxed then it is obviously not necessary to take the tablets. This is all quite logical, but it is using a non-medical frame of reference.

Whether or not the patient adheres to the treatment leads to the final outcome in the patient's learning circle. As Stimpson and Webb (1975) pointed out:

> The crucial paradox . . . is that in the consultation the doctor makes the treatment decisions; after the consultation, decision making lies with the patient.

Shared decision making

A good friend of mine, David Smith, who is an American Professor of Medical Ethics, found in a study of expressed consultation preferences that in the UK, the USA and Australia most patients preferred joint decision making rather than either delegating the decision to the doctor or deciding alone. Many subsequent papers have confirmed this view.

In 1990 Lesley Fallowfield studied a cohort of women with breast cancer who were treated by three groups of surgeons – one group whose policy favoured mastectomy, a second group that favoured breast conservation, and a third group that offered a choice of treatment. There was considerable psychiatric morbidity postoperatively at 3 and 12 months after treatment in all three groups, and there were no differences between the patients who had had a mastectomy and those who had not. However, the patients who were treated by the surgeons whose policy was to offer the patient a choice, including those who for clinical reasons in fact had no choice, showed significantly reduced anxiety and depression compared with the other two groups. More recently, in 2000, Brian McKinstry, a clever Scottish GP, showed video vignettes of five different presenting conditions to patients. He found that patients vary in their desire for involvement in decision making, and that this variation depends on the presenting problem, shared decision making being preferred for psychological problems, but the more ill they were or the more physical the problem, the more patients desired a directed approach. Higher social class and educational level were, unsurprisingly, associated with an increased desire for involvement. The variations were very large, making it imperative for doctors to determine for individual patients how much involvement in decision making they want.

Shared decision making is not easy for doctors or patients, but it can and should be achieved in the majority of encounters. This is a theme to which we shall return several times during the course of this book.

Long-term effects: change in health

We all try to make sense of changes in our health, and we tend to link them to changes that preceded them. For example, a patient with a bad cold may come to believe that a large tot of Glenmorangie is the best solution if improvement follows in the morning. Another patient may quickly come to believe that antibiotics cure colds if the doctor prescribes them with little explanation. Both of these learned beliefs are in the realms of superstition, and neither is helpful to either the patient or the doctor.

In chronic illness the steady drip of recurrent consultations may build up helpful or unhelpful health strategies – for example, asthma patients addicted to their inhalers, diabetic patients with bizarre dietary beliefs, hypertensive patients who are afraid to take exercise, and so on.

Look again at Table 4.1. What other superstitious beliefs can patients develop?

Somatisation

This final outcome of the consultation is an area to which doctors are now beginning to give the attention it merits. The word is ugly and obscure, but it refers to the tendency of patients to create physical symptoms out of emotional responses. This can be aided and abetted by doctors strenuously trying to create disease out of a mass of complaints, and a disease once created in a patient's mind is very difficult to dispel. Patients who somatise their symptoms seem to be less able to talk openly about their emotions, and often present with woolly, rambling stories linked to fixed, if odd, physical symptoms. They also tend to have an external locus of control. Most people have episodes involving physical complaints that are not explained by organic disease. Low-grade somatisation is common, especially in primary care (one in 20 patients), and was found to account for at least 20% of the workload of general practitioners in one study conducted in 2003. Effective strategies for somatisation are needed that are not too complex for general practitioners to apply.

Look again at the patient's learning circle in Figure 4.1. In what areas are your interventions likely to influence your patient's health understanding? Remember that your chance to influence this understanding will not arise very often. With some notable exceptions, patients do not consult with doctors all that often. This is particularly true of young and middle-aged men. This is, of course, one more reason why we have relatively little input into the health understanding of most of our patients.

Chapter 5

How you feel is as important as what you know

The doctor's circle of understanding

This is, of course, the other side of the patient's circle – meeting at the consultation. However, there is a big difference between the two. Most patients do not go round the circle all that often, whereas doctors are going round it all the time. I have seen about 6,000 patients each year for the last 30 years, which amounts to over 180,000 consultations. I wonder how many of these patients I have learned from? We are often told about learning from experience. Most doctors quite quickly gain a lot of experiences with patients, but how much do they learn from those experiences?

The doctor's circle of understanding can be drawn as shown in Figure 5.1.

Physical and emotional status

How we feel affects how we consult. If you have flu and still find yourself at work, it can be very difficult to think straight and to make decisions, and when it is apparent that most patients are feeling better than you are, some of your motivation will evaporate. It is obvious that we consult better when we are well, but many doctors, driven by inner goals, soldier on long after the point when it would be better for their patients if they stopped.

Emotional health is more subtle and more insidious. Doctors have a very high incidence of alcoholism, depressive illness and chronic stress disorders. The stiff-upper-lip, lonely, evangelistic medical credo

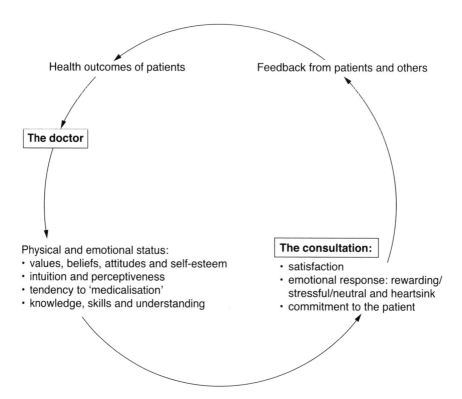

Figure 5.1 The doctor's learning circle.

forces them to carry on against the odds, rarely seeking help from colleagues, as this is perceived as a sign of weakness. However, at last the profession is beginning to wake up to the emotional needs of doctors. If you feel yourself becoming emotionally stressed, talk about it with friends, and try to seek help sooner rather than later.

Values, beliefs, attitudes and self-esteem

Like patients, we bring to our consultations a set of beliefs, moral values and attitudes that are derived from our own upbringing, culture and experience. These thinking and feeling patterns will influence how we consult with our patients. A few simple examples illustrate this point.

- If I am an atheist, I am less likely to suggest to a dying patient that they should seek solace in God.
- If I believe in the total sanctity of human life, I am virtually never going to recommend a termination of pregnancy or be involved in discussions about euthanasia.
- If I am politically left of centre, free market health service policies may be anathema to me, and I may work in such a way as to demonstrate my disapproval.
- If I believe that unsolicited lifestyle advice is an intrusion into personal liberty, I am not going to offer it very often, or if I do it will be half-hearted and only given because I get paid for it.
- If I believe that my job is to diagnose serious illness, I am likely to believe that my patients' ideas and worries are relatively trivial.
- If I believe that it is better for patients to be protected from the whole truth in serious illness, then I will withhold information.
- If I believe that the patients' ideas and concerns are important, then I will seek them out.

And so on.

Think about your own beliefs and attitudes. How do they affect the way in which you consult or feel about patients? Can you compromise from time to time? Can you justify your attitudes to yourself? Can you justify them to your peers? Would you say that you have an accepting attitude with regard to your patient's point of view and beliefs, or is it more a judgmental attitude which equates your patient's worth with their knowledge and beliefs, and places your point of view above theirs?

Our self-esteem is relevant. What is our status? How important is status to us and how motivating is it? Do we need to be powerful in order to protect our fragile self-esteem? Do you consult with patients in such a way as to enhance your own self-esteem, or is this not too important a factor to you? How important is the approval of your friends and peers? How do you maintain your self-respect when dealing with your patients? How do you develop self-confidence? Think about it.

Intuition and perceptiveness

These are both God-given and learned. Intuitive medical behaviour may be based on experience – an effective synaptic short-circuit – but some doctors are better at it than others. Usually the more intuitive doctors are the more experienced ones. When you are learning, do not trust too much to intuition. Go back, recheck, and try to trace the intuitive pathway until you can follow the logical thread.

Perceptiveness must be learned. Sherlock Holmes remains one of the finest role models, based by Conan Doyle on a senior medical figure in Edinburgh. Consulting with patients, looking, asking and examining them form the basis for developing your perceptive skills. Really seeing them, truly hearing what they say (or do not say) and understanding them and their context are the flesh on those bones.

Tendency to 'medicalisation'

Ivan Illich coined this deliberately ugly term to describe the medical tendency to organise vague symptoms into categories, and to label these categories and so produce a disease that can then be approached in the traditional medical manner. This tendency is particularly obvious in the medical handling of the everyday emotional trauma which all human beings experience. For example, unhappiness is a human condition, whereas 'depression' is a disease that can be treated with antidepressants.

Labelling people creates illness. For example, people who are found to have mild hypertension and who are told this fact suddenly have more sickness absence, have a higher incidence of impotence, cut down their participation in sport by over 50%, have double the incidence of panic attacks, and view themselves differently. This is *before* any possible drug side-effects are manifested. Think about this for a moment. This means that all diagnoses have costs. To suddenly turn a normal patient into a 'hypertensive' is not a neutral event. Such a patient's perception of him- or herself has been altered quite markedly for the worse. Therefore you must be quite certain that your diagnosis and subsequent intervention are going to outweigh the harm done.

There is also the medicalisation of daily living – encouraging people to consult doctors about the minor vagaries of life and health, a creeping stripping of personal autonomy, and the gradual creation of a society that is dependent on the medical professions for all wisdom on diet, exercise, lovemaking and everyday existence. In April 2002, a whole edition of the *British Medical Journal*, entitled 'Too much medicine', was devoted to the dangers of creeping 'medicalisation.' Two quotes from this edition are given below:

> If we choose to 'medicalise' the whole of our existence, we realise that life is a pathological process, a sexually transmitted terminal illness whose prognosis can be predicted at the moment of birth.
>
> (Michael O'Donnell)

> I don't smoke or drink, I don't stay out late and I don't sleep with girls. My diet is healthy and I take regular exercise. All this is going to change when I get out of prison.
>
> (Graffito)

If we as doctors subscribe either consciously or unconsciously to this widespread tendency, it will affect the way in which we consult and the outcomes of those consultations. *A medicalising doctor and a somatising patient are a bad combination.*

Constraints

It is not easy to consult well, and our modern environment can and does make it more difficult. Contracts that reward behaviour geared towards population health improvement strategies discourage the open, patient-centred approach. Time constraints multiply. The fear of a complaint lurks in every meeting. Continuity in general practice is breaking down. True advocacy requires access to resources, but these are often scarce. The weight of patient expectations can be hard to cope with, and the constant uncertainty of diagnosis and prognosis weighs on us all. But don't get too disheartened – there have always been constraints, and if you care you can rise above most of them most of the time.

Knowledge, skills and understanding

This is the area that is traditionally related to the medical school. It is for our knowledge, and the skills to use that knowledge, that the public come to us. We learn about diseases and about techniques to diagnose and treat these diseases, and we listen to aphorisms such as 'There is nothing more important than diagnosis, diagnosis and diagnosis.' We slave over sweet-smelling corpses searching for aberrant nerves, and we learn by rote the mysteries of the Kreb's cycle. We are multiple-choiced to the point of exhaustion, and we are taught to learn by an adversarial style of one-upmanship. We feel guilty about reading a novel because we should be reading medicine. There is so much that it is unencompassable, and if we are not careful, in all this knowledge we shall lose our understanding of people and what makes them tick.

We must use our consultations with our patients to increase our knowledge, to hone our skills, and most of all to improve our understanding of illness, of people and of ourselves. Then, with all of these strands of ourselves mixed together as our 'givens', we come to the consultation. There is an interaction, a conversation, some laying on of hands – whatever – but at the end of the consultation some things have changed for us as they have for our patients. Let us look at these possible outcomes.

Satisfaction

We all want to do a good job and to take pride in doing so. This affects how we perform. For instance, there is some evidence that doctors who have low job satisfaction prescribe more tranquillisers and antibiotics, and have shorter consultations. In order to derive regular satisfaction from patient encounters, we need to like what we are doing, have reasonably clearly defined aims, and obtain frequent, supportive feedback that tells us how we are doing and how we can improve. I suspect that not many of us receive much of that type of feedback.

Satisfaction also relates to several internalised goals and the measurement of our achievements against those goals.

> That was a good consultation because she came in very unhappy but I spotted that, I let her cry and then she told me what was really worrying her.

The goal is to increase one's perceptiveness in order to increase one's therapeutic potential.

> That was a good consultation because I diagnosed myxoedema.

The goal is to be a good diagnostician.

> I was satisfied with that consultation because I felt we really did achieve a genuine shared understanding.

Think about what some of your own goals are with regard to patients. From what do you derive satisfaction?

Emotional responses

Dealing with people who are seeking your counsel can be immensely rewarding if you find that your knowledge and skills enable you to help them. This can give you a buzz – an emotional high – that is unmatched by most other occupations. However, there is a downside, too. You will meet many patients whom you cannot help very much, some in great distress. Some you will meet and know from the start that the outcome can only be a lingering, painful death. This will be hard for you, and you need to develop strategies to enable you to cope with this emotional pain. Many doctors do this by retreating behind cold, professional veneers, sharing little with their patients, telling them less, and effectively 'switching off.' However, there are more effective and less drastic strategies than this.

Helping people to die can be very gratifying if it is done well, especially with patients whom you have grown to know as people. There is emotional pain, but this is tempered by the satisfaction of helping a fellow human being through those last days, weeks or months – sharing knowledge, showing compassion, alleviating pain, facilitating communication with partner and family, using other medical skills to maintain tolerable bodily functions to the end, and not deserting them. Unless they specialise in terminal care, most doctors do not see dying patients very often, so there is no need to develop armour-plated communication techniques. In the vernacular, 'stay loose.'

There are myriads of possible emotional responses to a consultation. Sad patients may make us feel sad. Michael Balint suggested that the way in which patients make us feel is a pretty good guide to how they are feeling, so if you feel angry at the end of a consultation, perhaps your patient was angry, too. Consulting under time pressure, as most of us do, creates its own stresses and frustrations. In a busy clinic, when you are already an hour late, nice Mrs Jones trying to tell you her life story can wind up your inner spring until your teeth clamp together.

There are also those especially difficult patients, usually frequent attenders with incurable problems, demanding that you do something for them. This group has been labelled 'heartsink' patients. Most clinics have at least one person in this category. Somehow you will have to learn how to retain a sense of humour and compassion, and to keep too much cynicism at bay. It is true that looking at the list of patients to be seen can, on occasion, produce a sense of pre-consultation gloom. This is one advantage of reaching consultant status – you can pass on such people to your juniors. There are some patients who would try the patience of a saint, and we all have to find ways of coping with them.

You will hear much discussion of 'burnout' and also the epidemic of stress affecting doctors. This is a complex issue, but from a communication point of view as a doctor becomes increasingly fed up and stressed they see more and more of their work as trivial and unrewarding, and a vicious circle develops. Interest in patients as people wanes, their stories are not listened to, their fears remain unexplored and surgeries become wastelands of sore throats and headaches.

Roger Neighbour, in his illuminating book *The Inner Consultation*, discusses ways in which we doctors can care for ourselves. He calls it 'housekeeping', the point being that unless we can keep ourselves in good trim emotionally, we cease to be effective with our patients and our personal life will also suffer. You should read his book.

Commitment to the patient

After a consultation some sort of bond will have been formed. It may be tenuous and fragile or it may be a true contract, with responsibilities on both sides. There has to be some commitment on our part or we fail as carers. Our patients certainly expect us to follow through and to be involved with them. In our learning circle, we shall experience many different levels of commitment. A few examples are listed here.

- The terminally ill young wife with advanced breast cancer. You have become very involved with her and her bewildered husband, so much so that you have given them your phone number to call you at any time when they need you. Now that is commitment.
- The pleasant but chronically anxious schoolteacher with increasing panic attacks. He rings you when you are very busy and asks to see you as soon as possible. You offer him some time when you should be off duty. That shows more commitment.
- There is Mrs Arthur holed up having her iodine treatment. She sends a message asking you to come and talk to her. Do you go? She asks you to contact her husband and explain to him what is happening. Will you?

We cannot commit ourselves deeply to every patient with whom we come into contact, or we would be swamped. However, we must give each of them a degree of commitment. It is part of our learning circle to judge the appropriate level of commitment we need to make to an individual who seeks our help.

Feedback

The feedback we receive from our patients is haphazard and highly selected. The happy ones come back, write us letters, send us occasional presents, tell us how good we are and make us feel good about ourselves. The patients we have been less successful with may never come back. They probably will not contact us at all – we may rarely be chastened and hear one of them discussing us in unflattering terms on top of a bus, but usually we just don't hear. This means that feedback from patients is very distorted in our favour. It is easy to spend one's life in a fool's paradise.

Doctors need unbiased, constructive feedback. The current outbreak of patient satisfaction questionnaires is in some ways improving this situation, but most of the feedback is general, whereas it is the specific feedback that we find most useful.

Health outcomes of patients

If our patient gets better thanks to our ministrations, that feeds back into our knowledge store, as does the patient who does not get better. On a mechanistic level we can learn from our various tinkerings what helps and what does not help. We often pretend to be academic, and we live in the increasingly oppressive world of evidence-based medicine, but most doctors will trust their own experience of 10 people on a particular drug more than a clinical trial of 1,000 patients. 'I have seen it before and know that that happens' is a traditional part of the art of medicine. This is not to deride the scientific basis of some of our knowledge, or to belittle the power of the double-blind randomised controlled trial. It is just to acknowledge human behaviour and the power of personal experience.

Table 5.1 What doctors learn from patients' responses to protocols

	Patient gets well	*Patient does not get well*
Doctor complies with professional protocols	A	B
Doctor ignores professional protocols	C	D

We live in a world of ever more numerous protocols and treatment plans. As is shown in Table 5.1, you may find it instructive to consider what doctors learn from such day-to-day encounters with patients.

For example, the doctor could conclude from experience with patients A and D that recommended protocols are effective, whereas their experience with patients B and C could shake their faith.

Given the variety of influences that determine whether or not patients get well, this feedback is extremely unreliable. It is essentially superstitious – the associations inferred between the doctor's behaviour and its consequences for the patient are not necessarily causal.

Every patient is unique, and this is why medicine is so difficult to teach and to learn. What works for one patient will not work for another. If we observe the outcomes carefully and develop our perception, this will feed back into both our knowledge and our understanding store and will increase our intuitiveness. What we have to take into account in this equation is not just the treatment we gave or the advice we proffered. We also need to remember the style in which the consultation was conducted, whether it was doctor-centred, patient-centred, relaxed, rushed, how the relationship was, and so on, as all of these factors will affect what happens to our patients.

Look again at the full learning circle in Figure 5.1 and think of five patients you have seen recently. Write down what the outcomes of those consultations were for you, and then think how those outcomes feed back into your 'givens' – the items listed to the left of the consultation.

OK? Done that? Then now it is time to look into the black box to see what the consultation should contain.

Chapter 6

What you need to achieve in a consultation

- You must know more about your patient as a person at the end of the consultation than you did at the beginning.

What follows is not the same as the traditional method of history taking. In some ways it amounts to the same thing, but it is a better method. The concepts are rooted in the discussions in the previous chapters, and the model works for all consultations in whatever setting. There are four main headings.

1 Discover the reasons for the patient's attendance:
   - understand the patient
   - understand the problem.
2 Share understanding.
3 Share decisions and responsibility.
4 Make effective use of the consultation.

To use an American expression, let us 'unpack' each task in turn.

Discover the reasons for the patient's attendance

Understand the patient

Before you started reading this book it may have seemed obvious in most outpatient clinics why most patients were there. Now I hope it is apparent to you that patients do not come to see doctors because they have liver disease. They come because they perceive that their health has changed, and they have a whole set of beliefs and expectations relating to this change in health. On the whole it is doctors who tell them that they have liver disease. So where should we start? The best bet is usually with the patient.

Listen to the patient describing the reasons for attending

Remember William Osler's dictum to listen to the patient because he is trying to tell you the diagnosis. The simplest way to do this is to let the patient talk, actively encourage their contribution to the consultation, and watch your patient all the time they are talking. Look for cues (both verbal and non-verbal) and try not to interrupt too much. Use your perceptive faculties to hear what they are saying, and try to pick up the message behind the message. We shall discuss some of the effective skills later in the book, but for now just think for yourself how best you would encourage the patient.

There are good reasons for letting the patient have a minute or two of relatively uninterrupted dialogue at the beginning of a consultation. The first is that it often *saves time*. This may be counterintuitive, but it is true. The reasons why letting the patient talk can save time are related first to the patient's agenda and secondly to yours.

The patient, *and only the patient*, knows the reasons why they have come to see you. If you start on your agenda too soon you may never discover the fear of cancer or the fear of the effects of expected therapy, but more importantly you may not discover what it is that the patient actually wants to know. You may waste 30 minutes testing and reassuring them about a normal cardiovascular system when their actual concern was about oesophageal cancer. The woman with the breast lump who returns after a positive biopsy needs to tell you her ideas, her fears and her expectations to help you both to plan the best management.

The point about you starting on your agenda too soon is significant. It is well documented that doctors make hypotheses very early on in a consultation – usually in the first 30 seconds, sometimes even earlier. Once you have made a hypothesis, for example, 'This woman has toxic multinodular goitre', all of your energies are channelled towards proving that hypothesis. There follows a rapid-fire series of clinical, closed questions directed towards that end, to the exclusion of a broader picture. Another hypothesis will only arise if your clinical search is sterile. You will gain so much more valuable information by consciously delaying making your first hypothesis for, say, just one minute. Try it. It is hard to do at first, but very rewarding.

Establishing your patient's agenda early on allows you to negotiate the use of time in the consultation – to agree on what will be dealt with now and what can be left for another day. This is a very important skill to learn early in your career, as it can save so much time and prevent so much unnecessary stress.

Always keep watching your patient, so that you do not miss any cues – verbal or visual. You do not always have to act on them, but ignoring the patient's cues will mean that you will be less effective. A cue is a signal from a patient to a doctor to respond. Cues and responses can be both verbal and non-verbal. Verbal cues may be simply what is said, or they may be what is *not* said and may be related to the tone of voice, facial expression, posture or actions of the patient.

Here are a few examples.

The patient with headaches may say 'My husband thought I ought to come and see you about these headaches I have been having recently', inviting a response to discuss her husband's concerns.

Or to go back to your consultation with Mrs Arthur in outpatients, you ask 'Is there anything else worrying you?', to which she replies 'Er . . . no, I don't think so', while dropping her gaze and nervously fiddling with her handbag. Do you take this denial at face value? You could pick up on her verbal and visual cues and perhaps say 'There is something, isn't there? Try to tell me what is worrying you.'

Later, while examining her, you ask about previous pregnancies and she says that she has no children, but you notice that her eyes moisten and there is a slight catch in her voice. Do you ignore these cues? Or do you say something like 'You seem a little upset – why is that?' or 'Is becoming pregnant something very important to you?'

As an example of a verbal cue that is not responded to, the patient may say 'It's my back again', and you only address the present episode, without exploring the previous ones implicit in the cue.

Reflection can be a response to a cue. For example, the patient might say 'and I've felt low this week', and the doctor might reply 'Low?' Equally, the same cue could be responded to by a later statement by the doctor: 'You mentioned earlier that you felt low. Could you expand on that?'

Other examples include the following:

- 'You seemed upset by . . . . Were you?'
- 'I noticed in your records you had . . . last year. Is that still a problem?'
- 'You mentioned your family. What do they think about this?'
- 'Now that was a sigh – what does it mean?'

Picking up on the cues that our patients give us is a skill that all doctors need to develop. These are the signposts to the hidden or not so hidden agendas. No general practitioner can hope to be effective or derive job satisfaction without developing an ability to use cues and having a sense of when to act and when to wait. This takes time to develop, and its absence is one of the commonest weaknesses observed in registrars sitting the MRCGP examination.

In a study published in the *British Medical Journal* in May 2000, only four of 35 patients voiced all of their agendas in the consultation. The most common unvoiced agenda items were worries about the possible diagnosis and what the future held, their ideas of what was wrong, side-effects, not wanting a prescription, and information relating to their social context.

Obtain and use relevant social and occupational information

Why not do this at the beginning, too? At least you can then place your patient in a social context and begin to know a little of them as a sentient human being with a home to go to and, if they are lucky, a job to do. You will need to elicit sufficient details to place the complaint(s) in a social and psychological context, and perhaps to gain some knowledge of the cause(s) of the problem.

You will also need to establish the effect of the illness on the patient's work or home life. We doctors often forget about such effects, but to our patients these may be the main reason for them coming to see us. A chain-smoking miner with advanced emphysema may be hoping for some more breath to allow him to walk to the club and to be able to climb the stairs to visit his disabled daughter. The fact that we may not be able to offer more breath, but we know his reasons for coming to see us, may help us and him to make a realistic assessment. We can then offer the help of other agencies in providing wheelchairs, stair lifts, etc., while not pretending that we can perform any magic.

There are two ways to look at this task. As continuity of care is decreasing, it is becoming even more important to find out this kind of information in every consultation. In those circumstances where you hope for some continuity of care, each time you obtain some personal information you can regard this as a 'brick' and over time you will build a wall.

Looking at video recordings of consultations, it is surprising how often doctors do not seem to be very interested in their patient as an individual. Patients come with a sore throat, an attack of thrush, or for a repeat prescription for the pill, and all that happens is a quick transaction. The doctor knows no more about the patient at the end of the consultation than at the beginning. If this is our regular pattern, who are we kidding when we call ourselves family doctors? Make it a rule to know more about your patient when they leave than when they came in.

Just obtaining the information is not enough – using it is the crux. For example:

- 'So how is the back pain affecting what you do?'
- 'You said that your husband was upset after your mastectomy. Tell me more about how this has affected you both.'
- 'You said things at work are pretty hectic. Do you think that has a bearing on how you feel?'
- 'How do you manage at home?'
- 'This has been a bit of a strain for you, hasn't it? So tell me about it.'
- 'Tell me more about some of the stresses.'

Explore the patient's health understanding

If you have allowed the patient to talk for a while, some of their understanding will have been revealed, but some will need to be actively searched for – their ideas, their fears and concerns, and their expectations. Remember what you read in Chapter 3. You might get an inkling about their locus of control. Or if you have studied neurolinguistic programming (NLP) you may have realised that this patient would prefer a particular style of communicating. This will take application and practice. You must take the patient's health understanding into account in enough detail to ensure that there is a reasonable probability that the consultation will be successful. Remember that the patient is the expert on their own life.

For example, in the case of a patient with headaches the doctor may say 'You have had these headaches for a few weeks now, and I was wondering whether you had any ideas yourself as to what they might be due to?' This invites the patient to discuss their health understanding with the doctor, indicating that the doctor is interested and concerned about the patient's understanding of their symptoms. In its most overt form, it simply requires the doctor to say, after hearing the patient's story, 'What do *you* think it could be?', or something similar. There are few situations where such a question, properly and sensitively asked, is not appropriate. (The obvious exception would be when the patient has already told you – for example, 'I cut my finger this morning while opening a can of beans'!)

If the patient said 'Do you think it's an allergy, doctor?' and the doctor replied 'Certainly not!' or words to that effect, they would not be exploring the patient's health understanding. If, on the other hand, they had replied 'What do *you* think?' then they would be exploring that understanding. Clearly this task has a large 'attitude' component – that patients' ideas are intrinsically valid and valuable in understanding the nature of their problem.

In the early days it is easy to be put off by replies such as 'I haven't thought, you are the doctor', and so on. These are untruths, as everybody has some health understanding, but direct questioning may not reveal it initially.

Examples of helpful questions include the following:

- 'People usually have some ideas about their illness. What have you been thinking?'
- 'What would be your worst fear?'
- 'What had you been hoping to get out of our meeting today?'

To return to Mrs Arthur again in outpatients, you might ask 'Is there anything worrying you?' Your train of thought is to rule out an anxiety state as a cause of her symptoms. Mrs Arthur wonders if she should tell you about her fear of cancer, but she decides that would make her look foolish, so she replies 'No.' This is untrue but well meant. If you accept this reply at face value, your 'history' will be the poorer for it.

Enquire about other problems

The presenting complaint may not be the most important factor to the patient or to you. The patient may be presenting with an acute complaint while also suffering a chronic condition – for example, an acute pneumonia in a diabetic, intermittent claudication in a patient on beta-blockers for hypertension, thyrotoxicosis in a woman with multiple sclerosis, etc. You must obtain enough information to assess whether a continuing complaint represents an issue which must be addressed in this consultation.

Now to the 'proper' doctor bit.

Understand the problem

Having discovered in the patient's words why they have come, you can now form a working hypothesis and start to put some of your clinical pigeon-holing skills into operation.

Obtain additional information about critical symptoms or details of the medical history

First, you must obtain sufficient information to be sure that you are unlikely to miss any life-threatening condition. Secondly, your verbal investigation should be consistent with your hypotheses, which you have now formed on the basis of information you have just obtained in the consultation. This part is well taught at medical school, but do observe how your chiefs consult. What history-taking short cuts do they use? You may have to learn how to 'take' a full history, but there will be few times in your career when you do not modify what you have learned to be more appropriate to the circumstances.

You must learn to recognise, from what has been said, any potentially 'serious' diagnoses. These would typically include suicidal thoughts in a patient with depression, malignancy in a patient with chronic cough, change in bowel habit, dysphagia or weight loss, and so on. You may achieve this by asking focused, closed questions such as 'Have you noticed any blood in the stool (sputum, urine)?' or an appropriate question about suicidal thoughts

'Serious' need not mean life-threatening. A child with a cough or otitis media should probably be asked about asthma symptoms, or about their hearing. A person with backache should, unless it was manifestly trivial, be asked about 'red flag' symptoms.

Assess the condition of the patient by physical inspection if appropriate

The examination you choose should be one that is likely to confirm or refute your hypothesis or any other hypothesis that could reasonably have been formed on the basis of the evidence you have so far. This can be a little difficult, as the more experienced and expert you become the more hypotheses you will be able to generate. A thorough and intelligent examination is required. This next sentence may sound like heresy but – whisper it quietly – some patients only need examining in order to reassure them, to address a specific concern. For example, consider the case of an anxious young woman with intermittent chest pains. The power of the examination and negative ECG is therapeutic, not diagnostic, 99 times out of 100. Most good physicians are aware that if they do not know the diagnosis after talking to the patient, the examination will rarely illuminate it.

Make a working diagnosis

In primary care, detailed clinical diagnoses are uncommon in the sense of the widely used disease model of medicine. The diagnosis becomes a flexible concept to allow the formulation of a rational and appropriate management plan. For example, 'Sore red throat for three days? Strep? Virus, patient not ill and not too fussed about antibiotics, just needs reassurance' or 'Recurrent headache with all the characteristics of tension in a chronically anxious frequent attender who will need some strategy or therapy to improve these headaches.'

In hospital, the disease-based formulation is more dominant, but it is dangerously exclusive, as has already been demonstrated. For example, 'multinodular goitre with hot spots needs more investigation and probably surgery.'

Doctors need to form clinically appropriate working diagnoses on which they can formulate further plans for refinement of the diagnosis if necessary, or on which to base a management plan for their patient.

Assess the severity of the presenting problem

You have to use some judgement here. The simplest example is triage – practised by battlefield surgeons and by casualty officers on Saturday nights. You will have to categorise your patients' problems into types with differing degrees of severity and then treat the individual problem appropriately. On a battlefield you would not treat a man with toothache; in casualty you treat the life-threatening condition before all else. In outpatients, the patient with long-standing irritable bowel syndrome who is cachectic with a knobbly liver needs rapid investigation for malignant disease, and in general practice the woman who presents with a sore throat, mentions her chilblains and only later casually mentions a slightly lumpy neck needs to have her multinodular thyroid gland considered in some depth.

Share understanding

Share your findings with the patient

The reality is that this task usually comes immediately after the diagnostic/examination phase of the consultation. However involved they may be, the patient usually becomes passive and expectant while waiting for the revelatory pronouncements of the doctor. It is a skilful strategy to keep the patient involved, use their own words and continue to use the RAM-like memory of the previous exchanges.

This explanation phase is the cornerstone of most consultations, and often arises very quickly – even too quickly for many doctors.

Despite the difficulties, you must always try to explain your working diagnosis, what management options seem to be appropriate and what the possible effects of any treatment are likely to be.

Tailor the explanation to the needs of the patient (sharing understanding)

By now you have got to know your patient a little. You should have a feel for the type of person they are, so that when you begin your explanation, you should ensure that your manner and language are appropriate to the patient's needs and that the information is presented in terms which they are likely to understand. A very common medical fault from the highest to the lowest is to cloud explanations with technical medical jargon that is incomprehensible to almost everyone. Don't do it.

Your explanation should be linked to the patient's beliefs, which you have already elicited. This does not mean that you have to adopt all of your patient's beliefs – some of them may be quite erroneous – but you must tailor your explanation to the unique human being who is sitting in front of you. This will make it much more relevant than the standard talk on hysterectomy or the routine explanation about irritable bowels. Consider the following examples.

- 'I know you are worried about the operation, particularly because Mum had such a bad time after her hysterectomy, but hers was for a different reason. You haven't got cancer like she had, and there is no reason for you to get depressed like your friend did. Has the surgeon explained what is going to be done?'
- 'This rash is called psoriasis, and it is caused by overactive cells in the skin, but it is probably not affected by what you eat' (having elicited the patient's belief that the rash was an allergy to certain foods).
- Another example is the common fear of a brain tumour in patients with headaches, and then tailoring the explanation to take this into account: 'I know you have been worried about brain tumour, but I think your other theory that it is migraine is correct, because . . .'

- 'I understand your concerns about the MMR vaccine. This is the best evidence we have, and there is no link with autism.'
- 'You felt that the new tablets were to blame for these symptoms. That is possible, but if so the symptoms will wear off after a few weeks.'
- 'Although you feel that any activity makes the fatigue worse, research shows that gradually increasing activity actually helps.'
- 'You mentioned migraine and stress. I think stress is more likely because . . .'

Remember that an explanation is a one-way process, from doctor to patient, whereas a sharing of understanding is a two-way process and it cannot occur unless personal details, health understanding, concerns and expectations have been elicited in the first phase. Doctors who are sharing understanding are also formulating management plans and strategies while they are talking and listening. The act of sharing understanding is intended to clarify, modify and tailor the subsequent decision, making it more appropriate. Much of the effective sharing will be in the emotional realm – that of wants, needs, fears and irrational beliefs. Unemotional logic is not the stuff of general practice. It is also important to realise that our patients' expectations of medicine's capacity to deliver diagnosis and cure will almost always outstrip the reality. This is a true understanding and not one in which most patients wish to share.

Ensure that the explanation is understood and accepted by the patient

Doctors, on balance, are quite good at giving explanations. The fly in the ointment is that patients are not good at understanding them. Watch your peers explaining to patients and ask yourself whether they are explaining for their patient's benefit or their own. Many explanations by doctors appear to be given in order to make the doctor feel that they have completed their own consulting process, and the patient is barely relevant. Ask yourself whether you are explaining for yourself or for your patient.

What you must do is to explain your understanding of what the nature of the problem is. At one end of the spectrum this may be too vague to be called an actual diagnosis, while at the other end it may be a clear-cut clinical entity. Even this is not enough – you must keep checking with your patient that they understand you. This is a process that requires considerable skill, and we shall touch on it again later, but be warned that a glassy-eyed, passive patient nodding obediently is not necessarily grasping every pearl of wisdom that falls from your lips. You must make some attempt to reconcile your viewpoint with that of your patient. What you are trying to achieve is a *shared understanding*, and this is different to a simple explanation. An explanation is a one-way process: 'I am the full vessel and I will pour my knowledge into the empty vessel that is my patient.' This does not work – it has to be a two-way process.

Work from the MRCGP Consulting Skills module (November 2000) has shown this to be the rarest of all observed behaviours, with less than 5% of doctors demonstrating it in three out of five selected consultations. This means that it must be difficult to do. So how can you make it easier? Here are a few suggestions.

- It clearly implies the use of a question – for example, 'Does that make sense?' or 'Have I made that clear?'
- Better still, try saying something like 'I know today's discussion has been complicated. Would you tell me what you are going to tell your husband (spouse/partner) about what we have said?' (think of Mrs Arthur).
- 'You may have found this difficult to understand. Would you like to tell me what you think we have agreed?'
- 'How would you explain your condition to someone else?'
- 'Is there anything you'd like to ask me?'
- 'What else do you want to know?'
- 'I don't know whether that makes sense?'

'Is that OK?' is not good enough.

Share decisions and responsibility

Choose an appropriate form of management

Your management plan needs to be appropriate to your working diagnosis. This is part of the knowledge and skills taught at medical school and modified by experience throughout your career. Your management should of course reflect a good understanding of modern medical practice, and this is nowhere near as easy as it sounds. Medicine is ever changing, the slavish demands of evidence-based medicine weigh heavily, litigation lurks in every decision and pressure groups howl their demands from every corner. Uncertainty pervades all decisions. You can only do your best, and you have to keep working at that.

Involve the patient in the management plan to the appropriate extent

Patients should be involved in choosing their own management as much as possible, not least because their cooperation will be needed for the plan to be implemented. Management options should be shared with patients and, where appropriate, the patient should make the choice. This is another phase of explaining and sharing understanding, but this time it is about management, and the dialogue must be two-way. You may initially find this concept uncomfortable, but it is likely to make you more effective and less prone to 'medicalise.' Encouraging patients to see themselves as responsible for their own health may alter their locus of control a little and make them more likely to request information, as well as to use the medical profession more appropriately. As discussed previously, not all patients will want to be involved, and it is not always appropriate for them to be, but more often than not it is. If your patient is involved, the risk of litigation and disagreement is much lower. Try to work on this aspect of communication. It is a fairly rare behaviour in young registrars who are observed consulting.

Sharing decisions need not be too onerous. For example, consider a patient with tennis elbow. You could say something like 'Well, you've had it a few weeks now. I think the best thing is a cortisone injection – it's not too bad, you know. OK?' However, this is not sharing, it is telling. Alternatively, you could say 'Well, you've tried the anti-inflammatory gel. I find physiotherapy works sometimes, or what about a splint for when you are working? They are often quite good. Or what do you think about a steroid injection?', to which the reply might be 'Er, well, doctor, what do you think would be best?' You might then say 'Well, it is not necessarily an "either or" – the splint might be a good idea, but physio or the injection might be worth a try. Do you have a preference?', and so on. This is a dialogue.

Other examples of this approach include the following:

- 'So what do you feel about the strategies we have discussed?'
- 'Would you rather start the tablets now, or wait a few weeks and see if it settles?'
- 'I could refer you to our counsellor, or you could contact Relate yourself. Which would you prefer?'
- 'Some people prefer to adjust their dose (inhaler) themselves. If I give you some guidance, would you?'

The extent of the sharing will depend on the patient, how capable they are of engaging in such involvement, the nature of the problem, and what types of option exist.

Consider the following examples.

- A retired science teacher with newly diagnosed hypertension might expect (or need) to be involved very substantially in a variety of options, ranging from lifestyle modification, through choice of drugs, to the frequency and nature of follow-up.
- On the other hand, a learning-disabled teenager with severe tonsillitis might not appreciate a discussion of whether to take penicillin for five or ten days! Here a simple consideration of whether to use tablets or liquid would be more appropriate (and more helpful).
- With a patient with tension headache you could discuss the treatments available, such as analgesics, relaxation techniques, referral for stress counselling, etc., and allow the patient to indicate their preferred course of action. The patient with a sheaf of

printouts of Internet articles about their condition demands a shared decision, and this situation is now commonplace.

How would you share options with Mrs Arthur?

The underlying idea is 'shared decision making', whether it is about medication, referral, investigations or taking time off work. However, it does have to be realistic. The doctor is the medical expert and the patient is the expert on him- or herself.

Make effective use of the consultation

Make efficient use of resources

Time

Perhaps the most precious resource of all is time. As Richard II said, 'I wasted time and now doth time waste me.' We must make efficient and sensible use of the available time and, if necessary, recommend further consultations as appropriate. The use of time by doctors is a subtle area of study. It is not the length that is so important, but the use to which the time is put. In general practice, it probably takes a minimum of eight well-used minutes to achieve a reasonable degree of shared management and shared understanding. It probably takes longer in outpatients, as the doctor usually does not know the patient at all. There have been many studies on time spent with patients in all kinds of settings, and the interesting fact that emerges is that the amount of time spent does not seem to affect patient satisfaction significantly. This fact should remind us that it is the use to which we put the time that matters. Some doctors can waffle away 15 minutes with no difficulty, while others can be patient-focused, enquiring and efficient within half of that timescale.

'To consult well takes time – this is now unarguable' stated Professor George Freeman and colleagues in their *British Medical Journal* article (2002; **324**: 880–2), although I could argue with this just a bit. As I have said, a good consulter will do more with the time than a poor one, and many can achieve in 10 minutes what a disorganised consulter has not achieved in 20. This is of course too subtle for most research. One quality marker has been that longer consultations contain more health promotion – well, hallelujah, but just a small dose of caution here. When the MRCGP examination piloted the consulting skills criteria, we found health promotion by doctors to be a destructive process in many, if not most, cases. To trained GP observers the doctor's agenda effectively swamped that of the patient. You may find it worrying that in order to earn more money in our new GP contract, we will need to practise this skill daily – thus more and more time for my NSF quality standard agenda and less and less time for what the patient actually came to see me about. This, of course, may ultimately be good for the health of the nation, though not for that of its Exchequer. Time will tell, but not in my lifetime I suspect. Will it be of any benefit for Mrs Arthur?

So what am I to aim for? Good investigative consulting and patient advocacy, or protocol-based consulting with cash at the end of it? 'Oh come on, Pete', you are saying, 'that's a bit over the top – quality is quality, there's a good evidence base and we're going to have to learn effective consulting that achieves both agendas.' Well, maybe, but where is the evidence that we doctors are particularly good at either variety of consulting? And we can't escape from the figures relating to compliance/concordance/adherence with medical advice, which remain low.

In the USA, paramedics see the patient prior to the consultation with the doctor, and often very comprehensive questionnaires are completed that can short-circuit or facilitate the gathering of information, if used as an aid to communication. Sadly, in some of the clinics I have attended, they often acted as a substitute.

Investigations

Any investigations that you order should be capable of confirming or excluding the working diagnosis. There should be no place for armfuls of blood to satisfy every whim of the senior registrar. Costs are important and should be justified in terms of the refinements that any results might make to the overall management of the patient. If a test will not make any difference to the outcome or the management of any particular case, it will be very hard to justify. Always ask yourself 'Why am I doing this test? Will it clarify, confirm or refute what I suspect? Is it really necessary? Am I doing it just to reassure?'

We often do tests just to reassure our patients that there is nothing wrong, but unless their true fears are addressed, diagnostic tests may leave them more anxious than they were before. Several recent studies have confirmed this truism. The usual culprit in cases of failure to reassure is poor communication. A survey of 5,150 patients recently discharged from hospital revealed that 34% of them had not been told the results of tests. In a study conducted by cardiologists in Melbourne in 1996, it was found that many patients continued to be anxious about their heart despite being informed of a normal echocardiography result. Furthermore, three-quarters of the patients in this sample were referred for exclusion of heart disease after routine examination for insurance or employment purposes, which suggests that unjustified concern about ill health is often iatrogenic. Thus it is clear that informing patients about a normal diagnostic result may not always succeed in reassuring them. Ambiguous or false-positive results may create or worsen anxiety. It is much better to get your patients' fears out into the open than to perform unnecessary further tests or make an unnecessary specialist referral.

Other (health) professionals

You must consider the possible involvement of other professionals such as nurses, physiotherapists or other medical specialists. Only make referrals when these are necessary and appropriate as decided in your agreed management plan with the patient.

Prescribing

The cost of drugs is forever escalating, and the burden on national resources caused by inappropriate, uneconomical and unused drugs is enormous. Whenever you prescribe, ask yourself the following questions: 'Is a prescription really necessary?', 'Is this the best choice of drugs for the condition?', 'Could I obtain the same efficacy more economically?' and 'Will my patient take them?'

This last question is relevant in several ways. I have already discussed some issues relating to concordance. Another issue concerns our patients' understanding of the tablets that they are prescribed. Side-effect leaflets are now included in all packs, but these are couched in such bald and frightening terms that many of our patients read them, become afraid and then angry, don't take the drugs and then storm in to see us demanding to know why we prescribed such a potentially lethal drug as ibuprofen. There is convincing observational evidence that doctors do not discuss the pros and cons of various prescribed drugs very often – at best it is peremptory. I am afraid this is another area that we shall all really have to work on with regard to our communication with our patients. We must take steps to improve prescribing concordance and, as you are now aware, this means seeking out our patient's understanding of the treatment and a reactive explanation based on that understanding. Explaining side-effects and the concepts of cost and benefit and relative risk is immensely difficult, but we have to do it, and with practice we can only get better.

Research in the area of prescribing can be worrying. Here are a few examples of the results of recent respectable study findings.

- When the doctor thinks that the patient expects a prescription, he or she is ten times more likely to prescribe.
- Patients who expect a prescription are three times more likely to receive one as those who do not.
- Prescribing antibiotics for sore throats has only a marginal effect on the resolution of symptoms, but enhances the belief in antibiotics and intention to consult in future when compared with strategies of non- or delayed prescribing.
- Shared decision making about drugs is very unusual.
- Patient satisfaction with non-prescribing is related to the resolution of their concerns.
- Doctors rarely discuss side-effects in detail.
- Major misunderstandings related to prescribing are common, and are due to patients not being able to voice their agenda about their health understanding.
- In cases of atrial fibrillation, taking account of patient preferences would lead to far fewer prescriptions for anticoagulants than under published guideline recommendations.

Establish an effective relationship with the patient

The word 'effective' is the crux here. What you wish to achieve is a relationship that helps you to complete the other tasks. You must discover the reasons for the patient's attendance, define the clinical problem, address the patient's problem, explain effectively, attempt to share some of the decision making, and make overall effective use of the consultation. How you achieve this is your business. You may well have been taught interpersonal skills such as empathising, eye contact, use of touch, etc. These are all very well, but if used unthinkingly they may just produce clones of slightly damp Methodist ministers who are just too warm and hold your hand for five seconds too long (apologies to Methodists, but I had to upset someone). We have all met lovely, warm, empathetic doctors who are frankly ineffective, and also come across some pretty unpleasant cold fish who are effective. It almost does not matter whether you consult in green spotted pyjamas wearing a goofy hat if you can regularly achieve a shared management plan and a shared understanding. It is the achievement that matters, not the means of getting there.

I am exaggerating, but not a lot. There are, of course, some styles of behaviour that are more likely to produce an effective relationship than others, not least a genuine display of interest in your patient as a fellow human being, but there is no one style that will suit all. In longer-term relationships it may be the build-up of mutual respect leading to trust that is crucial in a therapeutic sense. Even with trust there are problems, as a very trusting patient may stop participating.

Concentrate on your strengths and what you feel comfortable with, and work on your effectiveness. If you are consistently failing to achieve an effective relationship with patients, then some of the analytical methods discussed later in this book may help you to diagnose your problem and find an appropriate remedy.

Give opportunistic health promotion advice

There are some areas of preventive behaviour about which we as a profession are pretty convinced – for example, smoking is bad for you, immunisation is good for you, as is regular moderate exercise, and probably regular cervical smears, etc. Other dietary and lifestyle messages depend on your beliefs, such as the value of regular breast self-examination, cholesterol watching, egg eating and salmonella, and the legions of other advice in the 'Nanny knows best' style. You have to make the best decisions you can on the basis of the available evidence. The point at issue here is whether you should take an appropriate moment in the consultation to give such advice. Linking lifestyle advice to a current illness can be quite an effective way of altering behaviour. Just telling patients to stop smoking and giving them a leaflet will mean that 5–10% will give up – an astonishingly high figure when you think of how many patients you see. This is another area for you to think about. The consultation does provide the opportunity for such advice, but not to the exclusion of the patient's agenda. Butler and colleagues reported in the *British Medical Journal* in 1998 that repeated advice to patients to stop smoking was likely to be ineffective, or even counter-productive. They showed that intervention was much more likely to be effective if it was patient-centred and respectful of individuals' circumstances, attitudes and choices.

As I have already intimated in the section on time, it has become clear in the last two decades that this task, now an integral part of every GP's contract, has grave implications for effective communication if it is misused. It is very obvious that it needs to be performed sensitively and in the context of the patient's stated or implied wishes, and it must not be allowed to obscure the patient's agenda.

Examples of what *not* to do include the following:

- 'Let's leave your headaches and talk about your cholesterol.'
- 'Here's a tissue – now when is your next mammogram?'
- 'The computer says you are here for your BP check, so up with the sleeve.'
- 'I think smoking is more important to discuss than your legs, don't you?'

Safety netting

At the end of the consultation you must set the appropriate conditions and the timescale for your patient to return for review, in terms of their symptoms or some other parameter – for example, a falling peak flow reading.

Shared decision making: a recap

In the twenty-first century the goal of most consultations must be to achieve a level of shared decision making. Let me go through the necessary elements again. True shared decision making requires a partnership with your patient. You must establish your patient's preference with regard to the amount and type of information and clarify their wish for involvement. You must also respond to their ideas, concerns and expectations. It is now that you must seek to achieve a shared understanding and allow your patient to reflect upon and assess the impact of alternative decisions with regard to their values and lifestyle. You must share the management options, identify choices and, if necessary, evaluate the research evidence in relation to the individual patient. To complete the task you must negotiate and finally agree upon an action plan, and if necessary make arrangements for follow-up. This added burden on the modern doctor is onerous but, if done properly, hopefully enjoyable and satisfying.

With regard to what you wish to achieve with your patients as the years go by, here are a couple of poems to get you thinking. The first is by WH Auden, and was his description of the type of doctor he wanted for himself.

> Give me a doctor partridge plump,
> short in the leg and broad in the rump,
> an endomorph with gentle hands,
> who'll never make absurd demands
> that I abandon all my vices,
> or pull a long face in a crisis,
> but with a twinkle in his eye
> will tell me that I have to die.

The second poem, by Marie Campkin, is the chilling updated version for the doctor of the new millennium.

Give me a doctor underweight,
computerised and up to date.
A businessman who understands
accountancy and target bands.
Who demonstrates sincere devotion
to audit and to health promotion –
but when my outlook's for the worse
refers me to the practice nurse.

Chapter 7

Ways of looking at the consultation

The first problem with looking at your own communication with your patients is that you have to *want* to do it. Nobody wants to look at their inept, stumbling and wooden performances, do they? I mean, why wear a hair shirt unless you are a monk? Life is just too short. Well, to begin with you must – you owe it to your patients and, what is more, if you learn to look properly you will find it fascinating, illuminating and immensely rewarding.

Creating a climate for learning

Looking at yourself consulting is unnerving initially. Others looking at you can be terrifying. Why is this? There are several reasons. There is the fear of being found wanting, of being exposed, and of being attacked and ridiculed. There are certain taboos in our society about what one cannot criticise, car driving and lovemaking being the two most obvious examples. Consulting could be a third.

Our medical school training often does not help – we are used to a point-scoring, adversarial, one-upmanship style of teaching. You have to know one more syndrome than your colleague, think of the blood test no one else has thought of, and take pretty fierce criticism on the chin. Some years ago, a nervous young student was having the mysteries of a diabetic retinitis demonstrated by an aggressive and impatient chief. The student had not fully grasped the skills of ophthalmoscopy, but was desperately trying to maintain some personal credibility with his irascible tutor. 'Well, what do you see?' To all observing, including the chief, the ophthalmoscope light was now brightly illuminating a patch of pillow to the left of the patient's head, and it was obvious that the young man was not seeing anything of the retina. Gamely, but unwisely, he continued to give a fictitious description of what he was not yet skilled enough to see. The chief bellowed at him, 'You silly little worm – if you had an IQ of one less you would be a plant . . .' This form of constructive feedback is not likely to make us keen to reveal our innermost secrets to a group of doctors. So how can we create a protected environment? It's easy – there are just two rules.

Rules for feedback

- Rule 1. Good points first.
- Rule 2. No criticism without recommendation.

There you are – simple, eh? There is actually a third rule, which is *always obey the first two*.

Simple these rules might be, but that does not mean they are always easy to keep and enforce. Let us look at rule 1 first. I have worked with general practitioner registrars for over two decades, and these rules are foreign to most of them. So after they have watched their first consultation I say 'Great, OK now, what did you do well?' This more often than not produces a phenomenon I shall call the 'goldfish sign.' A glazed look spreads over their physiognomy, and their mouth begins to open and shut involuntarily, emitting no sound. Most of us are not used to recognising what we did well. Instead we watch ourselves with mounting self-disgust.

> Oh Lord, look at that, I missed that cue altogether. Gosh, I am glad my professor didn't see that examination. What a rotten explanation. I don't think I understood it, let alone the patient. She will never come back. I was just so awful . . . and then some wally asks what did I do well! I didn't do anything well! It was all terrible! Oh God . . .

Ah, but you did. You did many things very well indeed. You may need a little practice to recognise your strengths, but recognise them you must or the baby goes out with the bath water. Learning from watching yourself consult must be a building exercise, not a destruction exercise.

If you are watching with a colleague or a teacher, it seems to work best if you start the discussion. In other words, the doctor being observed should start any discussion with what they did well. It is often necessary to clear away matters of fact, but don't be side-tracked into covert criticism. 'Which drug did you prescribe?' is fine, but 'Do you normally examine the chest through the shirt?' is not. If you are having difficulty recognising your strengths, this is when your colleague or teacher can help. No criticisms should be made at all at this stage. Only when you have a thorough understanding of what you did well and the skills you used to achieve your strengths should you move on to areas where you think you were less effective.

Doctors are very good at being critical. After all, we are not stupid. The problem is that our talent for supportive, constructive criticism is often underdeveloped. There is no place for criticism without recommendation.

> Peter, I thought when you asked her if she was worried about cancer and she began to cry, that you might have helped her more and perhaps discovered a little more of her fear. If you had just let her cry for a few moments, perhaps touched her on the arm to show you cared, maybe asked her why she was crying instead of just carrying on a little abruptly. I wonder if you were afraid of the emotions she might release?

This is fine. I may not agree with all of the comments, but I have been given some positive suggestions about my behaviour which I can use or not, and the discussion can be an open but sensitive one in which I am not unduly threatened.

> Peter, you were a bit insensitive when she started to cry. You must work on that and do better next time.

This is unhelpful because I do not know what to work on. I am just left feeling vaguely inadequate.

A problem has arisen in some groups that use 'good points first' rules, in that a degree of cynicism develops. Over the years two useful terms have been coined that highlight this difficulty. These are the 'Blodgit', which is the standard unit of insincere praise, and the 'Shit Sandwich', which indicates that if you are not careful everything before the 'but what could you have done better?' question is bullshit. Only integrity, honesty and practice can get rid of this, otherwise the exercise will degenerate into a sham.

Start using the rules now with your friends, and try to persuade some of your teachers to follow suit. In my experience of groups there is sometimes initial frustration at the constraints imposed by these rules and someone will say in as many words 'Come on, Peter, stop pussyfooting about. Hit me with what you really think. What am I bad at?' The trouble with this approach is that eventually the teacher can relent and do just what has been requested. The result is obvious in the metaphorical sense. If you hit a human being hard enough they will always fall over, and that is what happens, and why the rules are there in the first place. Don't break them. Using such rules does not mean that you cannot touch on difficult personal areas and areas of special sensitivity. It just means that it takes time to create a supportive, trusting environment in which such delicate and mean-ingful discussions can genuinely take place to the considerable benefit of the learner, namely you.

Ways of looking

You do not need high-tech equipment to look at how you consult. For a start, thinking over what you have just achieved with a patient is useful. Being observed by a colleague who can give you supportive feedback helps, and all that needs is an extra chair. Psychotherapy departments are prone to one-way mirrors, although I must confess to never feeling comfortable with such a set-up. The disadvantage of all of those methods is that there is no action replay. The advantage is that patient consent, although it should always be asked for, does not need to be formalised.

The two methods of recording that are currently in use are audiotape and camcorders (either DVD or hard disk). Videotape is nearly extinct. Audiotaping is cheap, unobtrusive and easy, but pretty boring. Visual recording is much more stimulating – you catch the expressions and the non-verbal behaviour, and it is just more likely to hold your attention. However, it is more complicated, more difficult to set up, more threatening and more can go wrong. Having said all that, most families have now used a camcorder at some stage, and the technology is pretty familiar. Modern equipment is sensitive to low light, so will work in the dingiest of outpatient suites or surgeries. It is all colour these days, and all new equipment will date and (more usefully) time stamp the recording. There are still a variety of formats, which can be confusing. The smaller, more convenient camcorders are rapidly becoming solid state, and will then allow easy transfer to DVD and long recording times. This is ideal for building a portfolio of consultations, and such equipment is becoming quite cheap.

The on-camera microphones are now quite good, but if you want better sound quality (and it is poor sound quality that ruins more recordings than anything else) you should use an external microphone. Many hospitals have audio-visual departments that can help, and all general practice trainers these days have experience of regular recording. Many general practices now have fixed camera brackets in surgeries, but most will need a tripod. A wide-angle lens is very helpful, as many consulting areas are fairly cramped. Although you can simply double the field of view by bouncing off a mirror, you lose light, but modern cameras are so light-sensitive that this does not matter. The aim must be to have both patient and doctor in shot with clear facial expressions. If you can only get one clearly, go for the patient.

Simulated patients

If you ever get the opportunity to work with actors or health professionals simulating real patients, do take it. You can obtain really useful feedback from an articulate, non-passive patient telling you what they really thought about your strengths and your less effective strategies. The wonderful thing about simulation as a learning tool is the fact that in real life it is almost impossible to know what any patient's 'script' is. In simulation this is known, so you can see how far you got.

Simulation is also very useful for short-circuiting your learning circle, as it is able to produce particular patients with particular problems on demand. There are groups of actors in the UK, and particularly in the USA, who specialise in realistic simulation of patients. In the USA, some actors have developed the ability to simulate real physical signs such as peritonitis, and even tenderness of the cervix simulating ectopic pregnancy! Simulation may well be a growth area in medical training – it is certainly a growth area in medical examinations. This alone is a good reason for familiarising yourself with the simulated consultation.

The next assessment development is likely to be the simulated real patient – if you see what I mean – turning up in your surgery pretending to be a newly diagnosed diabetic. This technique has demonstrated in stark clarity that doctors do not do what they say they will do in examinations.

There is a commonly quoted pyramid of the assessment of clinical competence (Miller's), which includes communication (*see* Figure 7.1).

Direct observation is at the top, simulation is shows how, and knowing is a long way from doing.

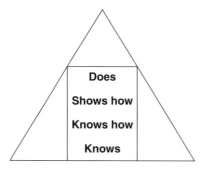

Figure 7.1 Miller's pyramid for the assessment of clinical competence.

Role play

Role play is do-it-yourself simulation and can be very useful. Unfortunately, most people come out in a rash as soon as it is mentioned and cannot be found for days. It has always seemed to me that this fear is misplaced because, so long as the rules are strictly enforced, role play has some safety valves built into it. The first of these is that it is artificial, and that is a legitimate defence for erratic performance, especially early on. The second is that we all vary in our ability to act, and being a terrible actor is not synonymous with poor medicine – the opposite also applies. The enormous strength of role play is the occasion when you play the patient. Here you can really put yourself into their role and begin to understand what it feels like. This is worth much embarrassment and angst, and you really must seize every opportunity you get, as it truly will make you a better doctor. Another advantage of role play is that it requires no technology, although a recording does improve its usefulness.

Real patients

On balance, most people do not mind being observed, discussed or recorded, but there have to be rules and respect for the individual. Patients know when they go to hospitals that they will be seen more often than not by at least two doctors, and often by a pack of them. This is no excuse at all for the time-honoured medical practice of then discussing a fellow human being as if they were an antique clock, with the occasional excruciatingly patronising aside. Patients should be involved as much as possible in discussions about their condition. Any detailed, jargon-ridden speculation should be continued outside their hearing. If any form of recording of the interview is to be made, written permission should be sought. The patient should opt in, not out, and have an opportunity to opt out afterwards. Visual recordings and audiotapes should be erased after the teaching session, and if they are required for a larger presentation, the patient's written permission should be sought again, preferably after allowing him or her to hear or to see the recording.

Patients are less passive in the less frightening and more familiar general practice setting, and are more likely to assert themselves by refusing permission to be observed. There have been many studies on refusal rates (which range from 1% to 60%), and the variables that seem to be most important (other than the patient) are the ambience of the practice and the way in which the message is sold. A gruff receptionist telling a new patient that 'Dr Tate is filming tonight, but you don't have to have it' is likely to elicit a much higher refusal rate than a patient who has been told when she booked an appointment that the surgery is being recorded for internal teaching purposes, especially if she is given a leaflet on arrival offering further explan- ation, including assurance that any personal examination will not be on camera. Curiously, the actual condition, including problems with naughty bits, etc., does not consistently explain patients' refusal. It is better to get permission sorted out outside the consulting-room in order to ensure that the dynamics are not upset too much. Patients do not worry unduly about being observed, and it does not change their behaviour in any significant way. In my own surgery, I had a moderately conspicuous camera *in situ* for several months – always switched off, of course – without explicit permission, and only one person commented on it in all that time. This was a young woman requiring an internal examination who, while in a compromising position, suddenly spotted the camera and said demurely, 'Do I smile now?'

Chapter 8

Ways of describing and evaluating consultations

In this chapter there will be examples of different ways of describing consultations, as a guide to help you to recognise your own style.

It is easy to discuss a recently observed consultation. There is usually some hot topic to which the conversation is drawn – often diagnosis or treatment or some peculiarity of the patient – but it can increase the learning potential of any observed consultation to work from a written description of the interaction. This can also then provide a hard copy of an ephemeral event. Such a description enables any subsequent ratings or judgements to be closely based on reality rather than the imperfect memory of distorted perception.

A consultation critique sheet (see Figure 8.1)

This is a useful sheet to fill in when watching most consultations. You will find it more useful to fill in those areas in which you felt you did well first, and then the areas in which you felt you could have done better. Using such a sheet allows you to focus on specific areas of your performance, and will help you to learn to recognise your strengths and weaknesses. When you start, concentrate on the first few headings, and gradually move down the whole sheet over a period of weeks.

Mapping the consultation

A map of a consultation is just as it sounds – like a road map, it can tell you where you have been, how you got there and where you could

What was done well and why?	How could it be done better?

Discover the reasons for the patient's attendance

- Encourage the patient's contribution
- *Observe and use cues*
- **Obtain relevant information on social and occupational circumstances**
- **Explore the patient's health understanding**

Define the clinical problems

- Sufficient information for no serious condition to be missed
- A reasonable examination
- An appropriate working diagnosis

Share understanding

- Explain the diagnosis, management and effects of treatment
- Use appropriate language, tailored to the patient
- *Use the patient's health understanding*
- *Check their understanding*

Share decision making

- Make sure the plan is appropriate for the working diagnosis
- Involve the patient in the management decision
- Discover their beliefs regarding prescribing and negotiate in a way likely to enhance concordance
- Prescribe appropriately

Effectiveness

- Use time appropriately
- Safety netting
- Develop and use your relationship
- Give opportunistic health advice

Figure 8.1 A consultation critique sheet.

have gone. There are many types of events that can be mapped, including interactions, questions, explanations, tasks, and so on. The original description of mapping consultation tasks is contained in the book *The Consultation: an approach to learning and teaching*, by David Pendleton and colleagues (published by Oxford University Press in 1984). The map that I shall demonstrate here is similar. You can, of course, create your own map to record those behaviours on which you are focusing.

The example shown is the map of the last consultation on a Friday evening (*see* Figure 8.2). The patient is male, 58 years old, and I do not know him very well. The detailed descriptions of the consultation later in the chapter will make it much clearer, but for the moment just look at the path of the consultation as demonstrated, and observe the movement between areas which occurs.

To use the map, watch a consultation and enter a cross every time you feel that a significant exchange occurs. Sometimes you will consider that two events occur at once, such as taking a clinical history and making an examination, or writing a prescription (action taken) and talking about possible side-effects (management discussion), in which case you should put a cross in both areas. The map is not a precise tool, but it will leave you with a reasonable record of the sequence of events. If two of you complete a map of the same consultation, the differences can highlight different perceptions and form the basis for significant discussion and learning.

Many consultations, especially in general practice, contain multiple problem presentations. To distinguish these on the same map, you can use other symbols or different coloured pencils. If your videotape does not have a time stamp, you can record the video recorder index numbers at points of significant interest on the map to allow easy replay. After completion of the consultation, join all of the crosses and other symbols together sequentially using a ruler. With a little practice, you can map consultations of colleagues while their consultations are in progress. This gives you a permanent record without technology, and prevents a lot of arguments about what did and did not occur.

Now that you have your record, what use can you make of it? First, you must be aware of what the map does not do very well. As I have said, it is like a road map – it will tell you the places you visited and the

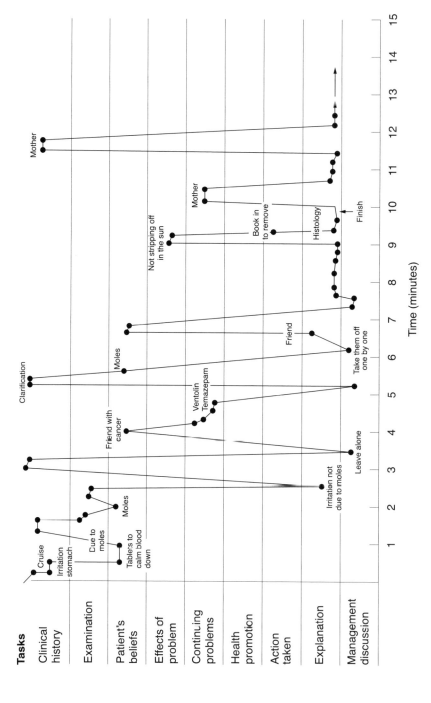

Figure 8.2 A consultation map.

ones you did not, but it will not tell you what they were like. Road maps do not tell you whether it was a pretty village or an ugly, run-down place – you have to make that quality judgement. It is just the same with the consultation map. Your map may show you spending ten minutes examining your patient, but you and your colleagues will have to judge how appropriate and efficient that examination was. The map only tells you that you did it, not how well you did it.

However, because of its sequential nature, a series of maps of your consultations can be very revealing, perhaps demonstrating the 'tomorrow never comes' syndrome. This syndrome is characterised by the response to a query as to why a particular task was not done at that consultation.

> Oh yes, sure, patients' concerns are important. I was a bit rushed this time, but I will definitely ask him next time.

A look through several more maps of your consultations may reveal that none of them have an entry on patient concerns. Tomorrow never comes. Used in this way the map serves as a guide to perform-ance by highlighting regular poor task completion.

The map will identify pivotal moments in the interchange which can then be dissected at leisure. The map as shown (*see* Figure 8.2) does not chart the relationship between doctor and patient – not because it is not important, but because it is very difficult to be precise about that relationship, and it does not lend itself to this technique.

The most effective way of using the map is to have a list of the tasks and the subdivisions, and to go through the consultation systematic-ally measuring yourself against these tasks. Do it in silence at first, and then start any discussion with the tasks which you performed well, and why you performed them well. What are the criteria which you use to decide what was done well? Learn to recognise your strengths. You can use the map to help you by writing notes on it at the appropriate places – little vignettes of conversation, significant statements by one person or the other, and what the problems were (e.g. 'sore throat, goitre, unhappy').

The map will, of course, clearly reveal tasks which were not performed. You have to ask yourself whether you can justify this. Measuring your consultations against various tasks a few times will soon make you aware of your style of consulting and what steps you may need to take in order to become more efficient and adept.

Look again at the sample map in Figure 8.2. What does it tell you? It shows that the consultation lasted twelve and a half minutes. It shows that the history taking included an examination and some of the patient's beliefs. It also shows that the effects of problems did not play much part in the consultation, but that there was a brief consideration of continuing problems, including the patient's mother. The explanation phase of the main problem (moles) seems to have lasted for about three minutes. The words appended to phases on the map remind us of what occurred, which allows us to review a particular area quickly if it seems helpful. Look back at this example when you have read the rest of the chapter.

Consultation self-appraisal proforma

I am indebted to Roger Neighbour for this idea. This method of describing the events of the consultation has to be completed afterwards, and can only be completed by the participant. You can do it from a map to jog your memory and give you the timescale, but it is better if the consultation has been recorded and you can review it slowly, stopping frequently.

Here is a description of the method, followed by a completed example.

Review your recording (or map) of the consultation, and stop the recording after each minute of elapsed time. On the proforma, describe or summarise in not more than 40 words what happens in each successive minute. Mention any significant remarks, observations, insights, thoughts, explanations or decisions. The idea of this device is to highlight your own perceptions of what occurred and why. This tool, unlike the map, also lends itself to exploring the developing relationship between you and your patient. The following example (*see* Figure 8.3) concerns the same 58-year-old male patient

Time (minutes)	Observations
0–1	I am tense and one hour late. He wants tablets to calm the blood down! I think he is anxious and I need to hear more. I let him talk.
1–2	He tells me about his moles. I ask a couple of questions seeking the cause of his irritation. I think he is very afraid of cancer.
2–3	He tells me more about his moles and I examine him – both a clinical and a therapeutic procedure. I tell him that moles do not cause irrritation.
3–4	I continue to examine him, get some more history and now he tells me about his friend who died from a cancerous mole.
4–5	I check his medication in search of the cause of the irritation. Temazepam rears its ugly head. We both note it and continue.
5–6	I pause, tap the desk, consciously stopping in order to clarify and review where we have got to. I involve him in the management decision.
6–7	I suggest, in a long-winded way, that in view of his concerns I will remove his moles.
7–8	He talks about his friend. He is quite frightened.
8–9	He asks me how I can tell the difference between a bad mole and a good one. I embark on an explanation.
9–10	I'm still explaining. It is rather one-sided. I do not check his understanding and ignore some verbal clues.
10–11	He tells me that for the past year he has been frightened to strip off in the sun. I tell him to make an appointment for a minor operation and tell him that the histology will confirm that all is OK.
11–12	He wants to talk about his frail mother. I am tired, reluctant to say too much, but share some of my thoughts.
12–13	He is kind to me and I feel uneasy. He lets me know that he is worried about his mother, but appreciates that there is no easy medical answer.
13–14	He leaves and I wish I had spent less time on his moles and longer on his mother.

Figure 8.3 A consultation self-appraisal proforma.

Are you doctor or patient centred?

	5	4	3	2	1	1	2	3	4	5	
I do most of the talking	5	4	3	2	1	1	2	3	4	5	Patient does most
I ask mostly closed questions	5	4	3	2	1	1	2	3	4	5	I ask mostly open questions
I am mainly interested in problems	5	4	3	2	1	1	2	3	4	5	I am mainly interested in people
It is my medical agenda that is most important	5	4	3	2	1	1	2	3	4	5	It is the patient's agenda that is most important
I feel responsible for my patient's problems	5	4	3	2	1	1	2	3	4	5	The patient is responsible for their own problems
I usually try to maintain, control and guide the consultation	5	4	3	2	1	1	2	3	4	5	I usually let my patient control and guide the consultation
I usually choose management options and plans	5	4	3	2	1	1	2	3	4	5	The patient usually chooses management options and plans
I believe in explaining	5	4	3	2	1	1	2	3	4	5	I believe in reaching a shared understanding

In relation to the above criteria, where are you usually on the scale below?

	5	4	3	2	1	1	2	3	4	5	
A doctor-centred consulter	5	4	3	2	1	1	2	3	4	5	A patient-centred consulter

Figure 8.4 What sort of consulter am I?

as shown in the map. As mentioned earlier, I do not know him very well, but I see his elderly mother regularly. This was the last appointment on a busy Friday evening.

As you can see, this is essentially a descriptive tool, but it forces you to collect your thoughts about the events, and with an astute teacher all sorts of topics can be discussed. The critique, map and this proforma are complementary. When you get a chance to observe yourself, I would suggest using the critique with most consultations, mapping a few consultations, and filling out the proforma for one or two of the more interesting ones.

Figure 8.4 shows another tool to make you think about your consulting style. You can't do this frequently, but it is a good idea to fill in this questionnaire at the beginning of your third or fourth year at medical school, in your first house job, towards the end of training and then later in your career.

In the twenty-first century it is clear that patients will have a much greater role in the assessment of doctors, especially with regard to

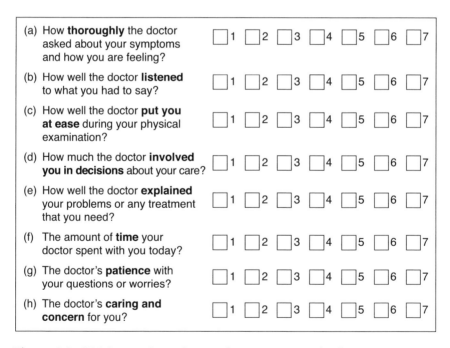

(a) How **thoroughly** the doctor asked about your symptoms and how you are feeling? ☐1 ☐2 ☐3 ☐4 ☐5 ☐6 ☐7

(b) How well the doctor **listened** to what you had to say? ☐1 ☐2 ☐3 ☐4 ☐5 ☐6 ☐7

(c) How well the doctor **put you at ease** during your physical examination? ☐1 ☐2 ☐3 ☐4 ☐5 ☐6 ☐7

(d) How much the doctor **involved you in decisions** about your care? ☐1 ☐2 ☐3 ☐4 ☐5 ☐6 ☐7

(e) How well the doctor **explained** your problems or any treatment that you need? ☐1 ☐2 ☐3 ☐4 ☐5 ☐6 ☐7

(f) The amount of **time** your doctor spent with you today? ☐1 ☐2 ☐3 ☐4 ☐5 ☐6 ☐7

(g) The doctor's **patience** with your questions or worries? ☐1 ☐2 ☐3 ☐4 ☐5 ☐6 ☐7

(h) The doctor's **caring and concern** for you? ☐1 ☐2 ☐3 ☐4 ☐5 ☐6 ☐7

Figure 8.5 GPAQ questionnaire: section on communication.

As a result of this visit to the doctor today, do you feel you are:

1 Able to cope with life?	Much more	More	Same or less
2 Able to understand your illness?	Much more	More	Same or less
3 Able to cope with your illness?	Much more	More	Same or less
4 Able to keep yourself healthy?	Much more	More	Same or less
5 Confident about your health?	Much more	More	Same or less
6 Able to help yourself?	Much more	More	Same or less

Figure 8.6 The Patient Enablement Questionnaire.

their consulting ability. With this in mind it is wise to familiarise yourself sooner rather than later with what patients think of your consulting ability. If you are already in general practice, most of you will have seen the General Practice Assessment Questionnaire (GPAQ). If not, you should go to www.gpaq.info, from which you can download the questionnaire in several different formats. When this book was first published in 1994, the thought of such a questionnaire being used regularly was a pipe-dream, but now it is an everyday reality. Figure 8.5 shows the section on communication.

A modification of John Howie's enablement score is shown in Figure 8.6.

In a paper published in the *British Journal of General Practice* (2006; **56**: 262–8), Mercer and Howie proposed a consultation quality index (CQI-2) as a measure of interpersonal care in primary care consultations. This comprehensive tool measures empathy, enablement, continuity and consultation length. This is a brave attempt to actually try to measure the humanity in doctors that patients so value.

Chapter 9

The magic move?

- Too much thinking can make us stupid.
- Remember it is what matters to the patient that really counts.

I have had a change of heart in the last few years. I now believe that most consulting skills come naturally, but that the attitudes and the confidence do not. I have heard sports coaches urge pupils to visualise the perfect serve or drive and then let their instincts take over. It will be clear to you that the first step is to think about what you wish to achieve (we did this in Chapter 6), but that is not enough, so in this chapter we shall consider whether we really do want to do it properly. If so, we must learn to consult intelligently, but is there also a 'magic move' to help us jump from the ordinary to the excellent?

Cleverer people than I have mused on the evolutionary merits of intelligence. We have found no fossil trilobites with large brains – and they were around for aeons of geological time. Then the amazingly big dinosaurs ate, fought and farted around (literally) for a huge time span without ever finding the need to develop mobile phones. So why in the last few seconds of geological time have we evolved intelligence?

Looked at dispassionately, our intelligence has not been an unmitigated success. We can destroy ourselves on a scale undreamed of in the animal kingdom, and with our capacity to meddle on a large scale we can now destabilise our planet even more quickly than the vagaries of the cosmic forces that surround us. Human scientific progress is now being made at a speed so fast that it makes no sense when compared with the relatively slow pace of evolution, even in human history. After all, since 'intelligence' arrived on the scene, progress has certainly not been relentless. Those wonderful and esoteric Egyptians came from nowhere to instant technological wizardry. The Great Pyramid is still literally unbelievable, the second one is impressive but not as good, and in no time they couldn't build them at all. They could still mould Tutankhamun's awe-inspiring funerary mask 1000 years later, but they carried on 'going backwards' slowly for another 1000 years until Cleopatra finished it off for good.

Ah, I hear you say, but what has all of this to do with communication? Well, my argument is that by trying to be clever we forget our instincts. The real problem is that we are not clever enough – our much vaunted intelligence is pretty superficial, and to understand things at all we have to reduce complexities to simple building blocks, thus distorting the true nature of the phenomenon. The number of blocks gets nowhere near the mystery of the Great Pyramid. An equation cannot describe the beauty or the mind-numbing infinite-ness of a Mandelbrot fractal, and a deep understanding of the Kreb's cycle does not help most doctors to cure anyone. Added to this, we become ridiculously possessive and overbearing about the small pieces of knowledge that we have gleaned. Consider the health professions. Cholesterol is bad for you, as is too much fat. Smoking is anathema and obesity is a dangerous state. All such statements have some truth in them but take no account of values, human instinct or experience, and the real truth is much more complex and multivariate, and capable of being viewed from many perspectives. Health messages become reduced to little more than slogans, and the complex instinctive nature of human decision making is not acknow-ledged.

We have evolved to make decisions about situations and our fellow humans almost instantly. For example, we are often attracted to another person across a crowded room, and sometimes we dislike someone on sight. We know from personal experience that our original impressions are mostly but not always confirmed. Human conversation is based on previous experience, unconscious obser-vations, pheromones, feelings and hunches, but most of our consult-ing is not, though it should be.

We all learn how to communicate from a very early age, and most of us are not taught in the conventional sense. When our teachers do attack us with subjunctives, gerunds, past participles and split infinitives (and tell us we can't boldly go), some of us are instinctively irritated, some of us make it a lifetime study, and most just put such grammatical pontifications to the back of our minds to be remembered in exams and interviews, but not important in our daily existence.

The point is that we are creatures with only a modicum of intelligence, but we do carry with us a barrel-load of attitudes. What is an attitude? The *Oxford English Dictionary* says that it is a considered and permanent disposition or reaction to a person or thing. I might quibble with the word 'considered', as many of the attitudes that I have are not considered, they just are – visceral, instinctive and sometimes clearly tribal. Some of them I am not proud of, so I won't tell you what they are, and I spend a lot of my life hiding some of these attitudes lest I end up with few friends. Are you any different? Alan Bennett's wonderful *Talking Heads* series allows individual human beings to display their naked attitudes for all to hear, and makes for riveting if depressing entertainment. Most human prejudices are attitudes, too. Attitudes are only very loosely related to intelligence. They tend to come from the mid-brain, not the cortex, and they are based on survival instincts and emotional feedback loops that are difficult to dissect and often not amenable to logical understanding.

The point I wish to make about attitudes is that they govern our behaviour. Your heart may sink at this juncture and you may stop reading because this point is so obvious – all that for this! But if you bear with me I would just like to point out that most conventional educational theory implies, and in some cases even states, that knowledge governs behaviour. The health educators are driven unceasingly (and fruitlessly) by this belief. I am not saying that knowledge does not change behaviour, but it only works when what is learned changes an attitude about, say, a procedure, a screening opportunity or a loosely held attitude (e.g. for or against the legalisation of cannabis). This of course makes the point that not all attitudes are equal – some are much more entrenched than others and much less amenable to the voice of sweet reason. Here again I must disagree with the *Oxford English Dictionary*'s use of the word 'permanent', as attitudes do change, but usually slowly. Now if we doctors concentrated on finding out the attitudes of our patients to the slings and arrows of outrageous medicine, we might be more effective in steering them towards doing what is currently thought to be good for them. Of course, the same applies to us – we have attitudes, too. When our own attitudes clash with those of our patients, we can only rely on 'professionalism' to help us through, followed by a strong cup of coffee and a gripe to our partners. Trying to find out what our patients' attitudes are implies that we are minded to do so – in other words, we have an attitude to an attitude.

People's attitudes are not necessarily what they say they are. This again is not a revelation, but an uneasy truth about a common lie. In the MRCGP oral examination, for many years examiners were taught not just to expose the attitudes of the candidate (e.g. for or against termination), but also to seek their justification of that attitude, the argument being that you can't really mark attitudes out of ten, but you can have a stab at rank ordering the justifications. This is not easy, and one person's justification is another's bigotry. Justifications tend of course to be post-hoc cortical intellectualisations of inherently mid-brain feelings. In the oral examination, all candidates without exception claimed that they believed in and practised the patient-centred method, and most could describe several consulting models and the concepts behind them to the satisfaction of the examiners. However, when the consulting skills examination came along, only 10% could demonstrate actually doing it in consultations which they had selected to demonstrate just that method. Here there is a breakdown in the theory – the stated attitudes do not lead to the stated behaviour, so the attitude must not be the real one, and the candidates are not telling the truth (remember the pyramid in Chapter 7). Are you one of them? Why do you find it so hard to do? Think about it now – put the book down, and think about your attitudes to patients and consulting. This is the 'magic move' – it is all to do with your real attitude.

Practising patient-centred medicine is in fact pretty easy if you want to do it – you just have to listen, be curious and participate in a dialogue rather than a monologue, but you do have to *want* to do it. Ask yourself, do I really want to involve my patients? If not, why not?

For years, communication courses have used models of educational behaviour – tasks, strategies and skills abound. There have been many programmes full of skilful simulated patients, hours of dissecting videotapes, clever skills training workshops, and – having witnessed 30 years of this kind of educational input personally as a trainer since 1976 and as an 'educator' contributing more than my fair share of tasks, performance criteria, etc. – agonisingly slow changes in actual doctor behaviour. Again, why is this? The simple answer is that the majority of the profession still do not regard patient-centred, evidence-based, shared decision making as worth the time and emotional effort to them, and if they feel like that, all of the knowledgeable clever teaching in the world is going to make very little, if any, difference. Is that how you feel?

In fact, the majority of humans, as I have previously intimated, do not need much teaching in communication. In my personal experience, many young registrars have become really 'good' communicators almost overnight in the sense of involving their patients, following a real attitude change brought about by an overbearing trainer or a realisation of the annoying consequences of failing the MRCGP examination. Of course they can then improve, and practise the skills until they become automatic and instinctive, but the first and fundamental step is the change in attitude. If we think about our attitudes, then our intelligence might be useful. Get the attitude right by thinking, then let instinct, experience and evolution take over and the results are almost magical. John Lennon was wrong – all you need is attitude, but it has to be the right one, and there is the rub. So the first step towards improving your consulting skills is to get your attitude right. Keep thinking about it.

Good consulting need not be difficult or shrouded in mystery. I suggest that you make a list such as the following 14 questions and pin it up in front of you. Let me highlight the second and fourth questions, about curiosity and what matters. If you are curious, it means that you want to know more – about your patient, their illness and their feelings. What matters to patients is the important part of their health understanding – a mixture of ideas, concerns, expectations and the reasons for coming to see you. The first time you can say 'yes' to all 14 questions, give yourself a pat on the back or, better still, a special treat. The second time you do it, you can allow yourself a small sense of triumph, and by the third time you will know that you can consult effectively.

Questions to ask yourself after the consultation

1 Do I know significantly more about this patient than I did before they came in through the door?
2 Was I curious?
3 Did I really listen?
4 Did I find out what really mattered to them?
5 Did I explore their agenda, including their beliefs and expectations?
6 Did I make an acceptable working diagnosis?
7 Did I use what they thought when I started explaining?
8 Did I give them the opportunity to be involved in decisions?
9 Did I explore their understanding of the treatment?
10 Did I make some attempt to check that they really understood?
11 Did we agree on (1) the diagnosis, (2) the management and (3) the follow-up?
12 Have I recorded the salient information?
13 Was I friendly?
14 Did I do this in less than 15 minutes?

Now a plea to teachers in medical schools, hospitals and primary care. 'History taking' is Victorian, patronising and, in most hands, communicatively disastrous. In an attempt to keep it simple, I only ask that every time a student or young doctor is asked to recite 'the history', the first questions are the following. What is the patient concerned about? What do they expect? What really matters to them?

Now let us go bird-watching. There are two species on which I would like you to become experts, so that you can tell them apart at a glance – but I warn you, it will take practice.

The first bird is the 'common nice mumble.' This is what many of us mean when we pretend to be patient-centred. It looks like this.

Hello, Mrs Arthur, I bet the traffic was awful . . . Don't worry about the thyroid gland, we will get it sorted for you . . . are you having a holiday this year? (while filling in a blood test form) . . .

> I bet your husband is worried about you (still filling in the form and paying no attention to her response) . . . Well, now, off you go and get these tests done – we will see you with the results soon and then fix the right treatment for you. It has been really nice to meet you, and you mustn't worry about anything.

The second bird is much, much rarer and is known as the 'lesser spotted empathy.' Here is an example of a young one – not in full plumage yet, but one day it could turn into a fine specimen.

> Hello, Mrs Arthur, you have finally made it to outpatients, so what has been on your mind? . . . Is that what you were worried about? Cancer like your aunt? I hope not, but you are in the right place for us to make the correct diagnosis and give you the right treatment . . . What do you know about the thyroid gland? . . . We may have to give you some radiation treatment with a special iodine. How do you feel about that? . . . I don't think that is a risk to you getting pregnant, but I will find out more details from my registrar and get back to you, plus the hospital leaflet to read. Next time we can go through some of your worries . . . There are those options we talked about – what thoughts have you got? . . . What are you going to tell your husband about what we have talked about? . . . No, no, that's not right, you won't need an operation at present because as I explained . . . See you in a month, hope you have a good holiday. Bye.

The common nice mumble is a robust bird, like the cuckoo, and can easily push the more delicate lesser spotted empathy out of the nest. The lesser spotted empathy also takes longer to learn to fly, with many abortive attempts and much flapping, and in its youth it can be a rather bedraggled, disillusioned-looking creature. But in maturity it is a beauty to behold. It is my fervent hope that as we improve the environment, this species will at last flourish and become the dominant one, but there is a long way to go.

Let me finish with a few words on how to recognise the lesser spotted empathy. Empathy, as defined by the *Oxford English Dictionary*, is the power of identifying oneself with, and so fully comprehending, the person who is the subject of contemplation. How can doctors attempt to do this without eliciting their patients' ideas, concerns and expectations? And does it matter? Oh yes it does. In an impassioned essay on the importance of empathy published in the *British Medical Journal* in 2005, Dr Craig Watson, an Aberdeenshire GP, finished with the following paragraph:

> In this age of science and technology and rapid access to limitless information, our powerful computers seem unable to calculate the value of what really matters. In defending the role, status, income and future of community doctors, science and statistics will no doubt play their part. However, because they form only part of our work they should also form only part of the debate. I believe it is time for our profession to assert the value of the art of medicine.

What kind of bird are you? What kind of bird would you like to be?

Chapter 10

Useful strategies and skills

- Good consulting depends on your attitude.
- Consulting requires skill.
- Skills have a purpose.
- That purpose is to achieve a shared understanding and decision.
- It helps to get the medicine right, too!

Even with the right attitude, sometimes our instinctive skills let us down. To consult well you need to be in the right mood, so the first strategy is to prepare yourself. You must try to generate some enthusiasm and curiosity for the coming encounter. Most of what follows is common sense, hopefully. Imagine yourself in your consulting room, rearrange your desk a little, have a cup of tea, stretch your legs and take a deep breath. Here goes.

Start by putting your patient at ease. Try to lessen their anxiety and encourage them over their natural diffidence. Some of us are better at this than others, but we can all improve – a smile, a handshake, an individual greeting in the waiting room, perhaps some easy social banter based on previous consultations, a little bit of personal warmth and good eye contact. Try to connect with the human being in front of you.

Your task is to seek out their agenda first, and your own second. When your patient arrives, greet them with appropriate warmth. Try to say as little as possible. Do not say 'What can I do for you?', and if you say anything, try 'Well now?' with a quizzical look and an air of expectancy. To begin with, simply encourage your patient – don't interrupt, but do nod, smile, look interested and avoid stopping the flow. This is harder than it sounds, as most of us make a working diagnosis within 20 seconds. With some of our regulars and in most hospital clinics we have made the diagnosis before they come in through the door. When you have made a hypothesis, test it, but be prepared to let go easily and form another hypothesis, and yet another, as necessary. Make an effort to generate several possible hypotheses, and try not to judge too quickly or by appearances.

With long-standing, difficult patients it can revolutionise your therapeutic relationship if you can clean the slate and start from scratch. You may be surprised by the results. This may be the most important strategy in this whole book.

Remind yourself that it is the patient and only the patient who knows the reasons why they have come to see you. If you start on your agenda too soon, you may never discover the fear of cancer, or the fear of the effects of expected therapy, but more importantly you may not discover what it is that the patient actually wants to know. Establishing your patient's agenda early on allows you to negotiate the use of time in the consultation and to agree on what will be dealt with now and what can be left for another day. It is a much more efficient way of consulting.

It will help you to rehearse the same questions that the patient him- or herself has asked already.

- Why has this patient come to see you?
- Why now?
- What has happened?
- Why has it happened?
- Why has it happened to him or her?

Put yourself in the patient's shoes as much as you can. This will automatically lead you to real empathy, not the much inferior product of sympathy with which it is so often confused.

You will need to listen with genuine interest. This needs to be real and not fake. Work at it. Actively encourage the patient to talk by nodding, smiling and echoing significant words. Show you are listening and watching (e.g. by saying 'You look sad today', 'That must have been very frightening' or 'How did that make you feel?'). The educational buzzwords for these behaviours are *'active listening.'*

Now comes the harder bit. You have shaken up your attitude (haven't you?), so now is the time to actively search for your patient's beliefs, ideas, concerns, expectations and feelings and the effects of these. Try to allow the patient to voice their real concern. This means more than just active listening – it means being interested and wanting to know. To be a good doctor you have to care about people, and if your patients understand that, they will in turn tell you what they care about. Practise picking up on the subtle cues – the sighs, the shoulder shrug, the hasty looking away and the rueful smile.

Roger Neighbour urges us to look for the *minimal cues*. Watch your patient carefully and listen to what they say. You must practise true seeing and hearing. Learn to pick up on the cues, both verbal and visual. This is the way into the real agenda, and if you miss the opportunity it may not come again. Watch the patient's facial expression, where they look, and what gestures they make. Do they make eye contact? Watch their posture, muscle tone and breathing. Do they look anxious, sad or angry? Think about their dress and their general appearance. Are they fidgety, relaxed or distant? What might Sherlock Holmes have deduced?

Really listen to them carefully. What does their speech tell you? What are they not saying? How are they saying it? Is their speech too fast, high-pitched, too slow, or does it have normal rhythm and modulation? Professor Higgins remarked that the moment one Englishman opened his mouth, another Englishman despised him. We learn a lot the moment our patient says something – their region, their class and ethnic accents being immediately obvious. We obtain further clues about our patient's internal thought patterns by listening to their vocabulary, figures of speech, metaphors and imagery, and their deletions, distortions and generalisations.

Linguistic experts have started studying the GP consultation. Professor John Skelton from Birmingham University is producing some excellent work in this field. His work provides food for thought, so look him up in Google.

Here are just a few examples.

- A *deletion* occurs when some detail(s) essential to a complete understanding are missed out by the patient. For example, 'I feel worse.' Worse than what? In what way? Or 'The whole lot are worried about Gramps.' Who in particular? How worried are they? About what in particular?

- A *distortion* occurs when actual behaviour and events are turned into protective abstract concepts which have no reality of their own. For example, 'I just lost my cool.' What is meant by 'cool'? It does not mean that you can shout and swear at the receptionist. Or 'I'm suffering from my nerves.' What does that mean? That you want more valium? That you want to see a psychiatrist? Or that the weekly trip to the supermarket is now a nightmare due to increasing agoraphobia?

- A *generalisation* means arguing from the particular to the general in a manner that excludes any possible exceptions from the rule they have made. For example, 'I hate doctors.' Does that mean all doctors, all the time, or me? Or 'I'm always getting headaches.' Does that mean every week? Every month? Every day? Learn to recognise the patient's internal search and don't interrupt. You need to notice when you have asked the patient a question which they were not expecting, or when a chance remark of yours makes them stop and think. Give them time to think, and don't continue with your own agenda until they are ready.

It is very useful to become more adept at demonstrating your grasp of the patient's perspective, as this can really help you to elicit their story. A good strategy is to listen, store up a few social and medical patient cues and then feed them back to show that you are truly interested and hearing what they say. This can be likened to using computer RAM, as it does require an effort of memory. 'I know you sighed early on when I asked if you had any children. Is that important to you?' Or 'I think you are worrying a lot about cancer, but when you say it is in the family, you must not think that all cancers are the same – most of them are not inherited. Was there a cancer that especially worries you?'

You will have to learn to modify your history-taking technique, fashioning it for the individual in front of you. Do not ask too many sequential closed questions, and try to focus on what matters to your patient and to you. Of course you must examine thoroughly but appropriately. This may mean not at all, but don't skimp on necessary examinations because of time pressures. Examinations are a good opportunity to learn things about our patients – and not just that they may have a large liver or an irregular heartbeat. The laying on of hands allows people to talk about deeper fears, and you may find that this phase of the consultation is often the most illuminating of all.

Now think about the beginning again.

Learn to speak the patient's language. Do not talk down to them, and avoid using jargon. This implies that we have a feel for the patient's language in the first place – you have to work at that. A weekend on a neurolinguistic programming course might help. Patronising 'doctor speak' should be a form of communication that died with the last century, but that may be wishful thinking, as jargon is so much ingrained in doctors that we often don't realise what is jargon to our patients. Keep monitoring your performance and pick out the words and sentences that need translating. You will find that watching recordings of the consultation with the patient can be particularly illuminating in this area.

A good rule is to tell yourself that, at the beginning, the patient is always right – and please remember to let the patient go first. Don't start with a question like 'How's your back?' Beginnings are very important and will affect the course of the whole meeting, so start open, not closed, and think of the difference between 'Hello, well now?', with a smile and a raised eyebrow, and 'It's your blood pressure, isn't it? Up with the sleeve.' Even the standard opening of 'Hello, what can I do for you?' is controlling, as it implies an action. You may think that this is nit-picking, but do experiment with the effects of various opening gambits. As with chess, you can win or lose the consultation in the first few exchanges.

Practise actively encouraging your patient to talk. Nod, smile and echo significant words. Repeat tentatively, in your own words, your understanding of their story. Reflect back in the patient's own words, not only to show that you understand, but also to enable them to hear and understand their own meaning. Try again if you don't seem to be getting anywhere.

You can try making statements which make good questions. For example, 'I was wondering whether . . .', 'Sometimes I find . . .', 'It occurred to me that . . .', 'My friend John . . .', 'Some people . . .', 'I've known cases where . . .', 'I had a patient once . . .', and so on. Concentrate on asking *open* questions – they are useful for finding out about patients' beliefs. Such questions cannot be answered with a simple yes or no. For example, 'Tell me about . . .', 'What is it like?', 'What are you worried about?', and so on.

The history taking that you have laboriously learned teaches you to ask closed questions, which are useful for obtaining and classifying facts, and for pattern recognition. They are not helpful for eliciting beliefs and feelings, as they tend to increase doctor control and they can only be answered very specifically, often with only a simple yes or no. For example, 'Is it painful?' or 'Are your waterworks all right?' (one of the worst medical euphemisms!).

You are now in the swing of things, so give your patient some encouragement, such as 'Go on' or 'Tell me more', which is the best directive I have ever found – patients always do tell you more. Eye contact and nodding encourage the patient to continue. If you find that your patient will not leave, it may be because you are still fixing them with your gaze and nodding benignly, so they get the message that you wish them to continue talking. Echoing is a good technique for encouraging patients to continue their narrative. This means repeating back the last few words of their sentence when they pause, to encourage further revelations. For example, 'Your mother?', 'Afraid?', and so on. You will need to pick up on the cues to do this.

Check what the patient has said. This can be done by giving them your interpretation of their story, thus enabling them to correct any misunderstanding and embellish the story further. This is a good technique, often used by doctors with a military bent. Explain why you are asking a question. This can stimulate unexpected responses. For example, 'The reason I asked about wind and bloating was that I was wondering about irritable bowel syndrome.' 'Oh, my sister's got that, and she said that's what I've got, but my mother reckons it's an ulcer.' Or, of course, there is the studied use of silence. This is often frightening to young doctors who, every time there is a pause, feel uncomfortable and duty-bound to say something, however inane. Try allowing pauses. The patient will invariably fill them if you wait long enough.

That is a lot to digest. Another truth may have dawned on you. You will need to practise, watch yourself, get some feedback, and practise again. Good consulting takes a lot of practice, but like doing anything skilful well, it is worth it in the long run, and the long run is your medical career.

The second half of the encounter

At this stage I should perhaps remind you that this is a book for doctors. Good communication skills and bad medicine are sadly increasingly common bedfellows – don't forget the science that you have been taught. This book is about communicating that hard-learned science effectively, so by this stage of the consultation I hope you have got the medical content right. If so, now you must learn how to negotiate with the patient.

The doctor should go first. You have to outline your position and your reasons. Try thinking aloud, and state your position. Be honest. Give the patient a few choices. Ask them what they think. Reinforce their good ideas and counter the bad ones, but be careful what you say. For example, 'Don't worry' means that worrying is an option, 'Won't' means might, 'Can't' means could and 'Shouldn't' means probably will. Use questions as statements. For example, 'Do you ever think you'll come off the tranquillisers?'

Again remember to watch the patient's internal search. If you do not see the patient looking as if they accept what you say, continue to negotiate. Watch for 'non-verbal leakage.' This may sound like a pool of muddy water forming round your patient, but it is actually the discrepancy between what your patient says and what their non-verbal behaviour is indicating. For example, 'No, I'm not depressed', while sitting with shoulders slumped, a sad fixed expression and exuding gloom. Or 'Yes, I will probably try the tablets', while break-ing eye contact and squirming in the chair. You have to act on these cues in order to be effective. For example, 'I know you say you are not depressed, but you do look it to me. Are you sure there isn't some-thing I can help with?'

You must try to involve your patients in the decision making. This may mean countering their fallacious arguments and erroneous beliefs, and reinforcing those beliefs that are helpful to the outcome. Try to foster patient autonomy and increase patient self-reliance.

Remember that you are more powerful than you think you are, so use your power carefully (*see* Chapter 2). For example, should you sit behind the desk instead of to one side? Should you fill your consulting-room with potentially frightening medical paraphernalia? Do not let your personal attitudes intrude too much, even though you are now aware that they are ultimately guiding your actions. You must be prepared on occasion to admit to uncertainty, and this may not be easy for either you or your patient. Uncertainty is all-pervading – it is the worm in the apple of perfection. Your inner self is always in doubt, but this is the truth about being a doctor. Develop your humanity and learn to realise that uncertainty comes with the territory.

You can use shepherding techniques. For example, if you do not want the patient to go to an osteopath, you can call him 'a bloke that tweaks backs for £50 a time.' Or if you do wish the patient to go, the osteopath becomes 'a colleague with more training in manipulation than me.' Another steering method is to use presuppositions such as 'Do you think you will find it easier to stop smoking all at once or to gradually cut down over a fortnight?' Or use the 'My friend John technique.' For example, 'I remember someone else who did what you are thinking of and found out the hard way . . .'.

Learn to use appropriate delivery, which is how you say something, not what. Start by breaking information down into manageable segments. Keep pausing and checking. Is the patient following what you are saying? Pace (the speed of delivery) is important. Try to match the patient's rate of speech. Eye contact is important. Keep watching for those minimal cues. Try to match the patient's language of self-expression. For example, 'You said you were "absolutely knackered." Don't worry, an operation like you have just had makes you feel that way.'

Think about reframing statements/questions to alter the perspective. For example, a three-year-old boy who is brought to see you because he 'wilfully' scratched his baby sister's face could easily be labelled 'attention-seeking', which could make things worse. What if he were labelled 'attention-needing'? Framing is a commonly used technique for selling treatments.

Remember that understanding of the words 'common', 'possible' and 'rare' can vary, and the use of percentages or other figures may be interpreted in very different ways. For example, patients are more likely to take a treatment such as simvastatin if they are told that it will reduce their risk of having another heart attack by a third than if they are told that it will reduce their actual risk from 12% to 8%. They will be even less accepting if they are told that the number of patients who would need to be treated for ten years in order to prevent one attack is 25. The important task is to convey such information in ways that are meaningful to the individual patient while not manipulating the message too disingenuously. This is an area of intense research, and the reading list at the end of the book might be helpful. There is a rash of decision-making aids appearing, and their quality varies enormously.

At this juncture, a word of caution should be given about a ghastly new verb that has crept into the medical vocabulary, namely consent, as in 'Go and consent Mrs Arthur for the ^{131}I treatment.' This is a doctor-centred behaviour and bears no relationship to the true spirit of informed consent. Informed consent is a two-way process, based on a shared understanding, checked by you, and a true involvement in management with genuine option sharing.

Take a breather at this stage of the chapter.

Now think about practising the second half of the consultation. It is my experience that enlightenment does not come all at once to most of us. Getting the first half of the consultation right will give you the springboard to perform the second half well, but the tasks and skills involved are very different. If you are a golfer it is the difference between driving and round-the-green play – all part of the same game, but very different actions are required.

Just as an exercise let us change tack for a while and think about those really difficult areas that involve trying to change our patients' entrenched and unhealthy behaviours. The GP contract and Quality Outcomes Framework (QOF) are designed to ensure that we make our patients give up the fags, lose the flab, get fitter or even take the tablets that they should be taking. The Government is clear that this is our responsibility. I think they are wrong, but how can we at least put our patients on the right track? Here are four linked strategies to think about.

- *Make things easy.* People are more likely to do things if there are fewer things to do, if they fit in with their existing lifestyle and if they have the necessary resources.
- *Think of the context.* People are more likely to do things if they do them with other people, if they are reminded at the time to do them, if they know someone might be likely to check to see whether they have done them, and if the people with whom they live and work are willing to help them.
- *Think of the patient's perceptions.* People are more likely to do things that seem important, and when they understand why they should do them and how to do them. If they really believe in your advice, they will follow it, and they are more likely to do things if their anxiety level is raised moderately but not too high.
- *Think of the relationship.* People are more likely to do things if they have helped to decide that it would be beneficial, if they have promised to do these things and if they have faith in you as their doctor, especially if they think that you like and respect them, and if they are rewarded for doing these things.

Now let us go back to the second half of the consultation and think about the crucial explanation phase. Remember that this book is about learning to share in the consultation, and the goal is to reach a shared understanding and a shared decision with your patient. This is a significant step further than a simple explanation.

First you *must* elicit the patient's beliefs. You cannot share unless you have something to share. This sounds breathtakingly obvious, but many doctors who are observed in the MRCGP examination are not actually doing it. You have to recognise that the whole consultation, particularly the process of eliciting, organising and reflecting the information that the patient gives you, is an experience from which the patient can learn – as can you. You can practise translating and sharing your medical knowledge honestly and with respect for the patient. This means maintaining or enhancing your patient's autonomy by respecting and not patronising him or her.

Here we move to a higher level of skilfulness. Try to clarify how much information your patient actually wants. This needs practice. It also means encouraging the patient to ask questions and to be involved. It is a good idea not to reassure the patient too soon, as this can be interpreted as rejection or a lack of knowledge. Bear in mind that while an explanation is a one-way process, the goal is a shared understanding, which is a two-way behaviour.

Practise presenting information without using jargon, use instead short words and sentences as specifically as possible. Remember that the order in which information is given is important. Patients recall best what they are told first. Repeat important pieces of information. A good technique to learn and practise is 'explicit categorisation.' For example, 'I am going to tell you what I think is wrong, what I expect to happen, and which treatment I suggest.' Again this may seem a bit military, but it is very effective. Get into the habit of using leaflets, tapes, DVDs, websites, etc. Read or listen to them first, as you may find that you disagree with them vehemently. Ideally, write them yourself.

Actively encourage feedback, check your attitude again, and regularly check your patient's understanding, not least because it will probably increase your own. It is bad practice to give too much information, and don't get carried away by your own verbosity. A patient staring out of the window at the squirrels is a sure sign that you have gone on too long.

When negotiating about treatment, specific questions are helpful. For example, 'How have you been using your medication?', 'Tell me when you take it' and 'What do you find the problems with the treatment are?' A word of warning, though. 'Why' questions tend to put patients on the defensive, and there is a tendency to invent reasons, such as the response to 'Why have you stopped the treatment?'

You will find that it will help to (metaphorically) climb a few steps down from your pedestal – in other words, try not to be too distanced from your patient because of your need to be professional. Remember to use similar phrases to the patient, and some of their own descriptions, and you will find it instructive (and sometimes cathartic) to share a little of yourself from time to time. For example, 'I had a heart operation and it shook me up' or 'Migraines are bloody awful, aren't they?'

It will help the whole process if you can demonstrate some understanding and empathy. Empathy is a much abused concept. The idea is to identify mentally with the patient and so fully comprehend them. This is fine so long as you realise it is only an aim that can help you to communicate with your patient. It may be impossible to empathise fully with someone, and you will find some groups especially difficult. For example, how can middle-class GPs really empathise with drug-abusing teenagers? We can be compassionate and we can care for them, but the vast majority of us will be unable to truly empathise with them, yet at least we can try to understand. Remember the rare bird, the 'lesser spotted empathy' – you are trying to be that bird, not the 'common nice mumble.' You must be prepared to back down.

Achieving a shared understanding does not mean always getting the patient to agree with you. It means that in order to achieve a genuine sharing you may have to agree with them. This may make you uneasy, but try to keep a dialogue going. You cannot share with a monologue.

Now let us recap some of the essentials.

- Determine the reasons for the patient's attendance at the outset. This then allows you both to set the agenda – that is, what you will cover today and what can be reasonably left for another occasion. This is a genuinely time-conserving strategy.
- Determine the patient's own ideas, concerns and expectations before you attempt an explanation. In this way you will reduce the risk of a 'dysfunctional' consultation, and the explanation will become tailored to that individual patient.
- Use each consultation as part of a learning circle. Some tasks can be achieved over a series of consultations. The adoption of these methods may also change patients' expectations about the appropriate use of time and resources.

Remember that there are other things to do as well. In all of this communicating you will need to record information (both clinical and patient-centred) effectively. This is another skill that needs much practice.

To be an effective physician, you will need to obtain as much information as possible on the availability of resources. Try not to prescribe prematurely, expensively or inappropriately. Another task is to help the patient to appreciate the costs and benefits of concordance and non-concordance. It will benefit both you and the patient to keep the treatment as simple as possible, and remember to share management strategies and decisions. The human capacity for self-repair should also encourage you to bear in mind the adage 'Do as much nothing as possible.'

To use time effectively, all of these skills need to be practised and honed. Self-observation is essential, and peer observation is very helpful. The skills of practice and hospital management, although beyond the scope of this book, are very important.

Here are a few tips and thoughts about general communication skills. Some studies have shown that a female style of communication results in more sharing and better outcomes. The good news for men is that they are just as likely as women to be able to demonstrate a patient-centred approach in observed recordings. This suggests that patient-centred medicine is not a natural communication gift, and must be learned by both sexes.

You can learn the skills of appropriate control, including the judicious use of doctor authority to control speech flow, and the appropriate use of negative non-verbal behaviour (*not* looking at the patient will tend to staunch the flow). Closing the patient's notes can signal the end of the consultation. Wearing a dinner-jacket tends to speed patients up a bit, but cannot be used too often. Standing up and holding the door open will stop all but the most dedicatedly self-obsessed. Removing the chair is a last resort. Feigning a fit is a desperation measure.

At the strategic level you, the doctor, should strive to create an environment that facilitates the exchange of information – for example, seating position, not having a big chair for the doctor and a small chair for the patient, ambience, accessibility, dress, décor, and so on. As I have said, be friendly and attentive, and adopt an informal style. However, be wary of the overuse of first names – it is easy to be patronising. The 'I am Lulu, fly me' style that is now universal in NHS wards is not always appropriate for complex doctor–patient interactions. After a while it is not unreasonable to ask your patient if they mind being called by their first name. Many patients quite like being addressed in this way but will never call you by yours. However, beware the patient's notes in this context, as using the first name indicated is fraught with dangers. For example, a Mr Cyril Blodwin may hate being called Cyril, and when with friends will only answer to Jack, so by not checking you may have been blithely annoying him for a decade.

It helps to use plural pronouns to indicate partnership. For example, 'I hope you agree. Shall we meet again in two weeks to see how you are getting on?' Use self-disclosure to establish trust and common ground. For example, 'Yes, I know you must be frightened. I am terrified of the dentist.' Make comments that are provisional rather than dogmatic. For example, 'I think your blood pressure probably needs treatment. Here is a leaflet to read. I would like you to come back to discuss the treatment and what you think about it' is preferable to 'Your blood pressure is up. Take these tablets – the nurse will explain.'

Try to respond descriptively, not judgementally. For example, on being asked the question 'What about my knees, doctor?', the response 'I think you have some wear and tear, possibly a little early arthritis' is OK, but 'You're too fat and that's why you have knee pain' is a bit bald – dress up the message. Make comments that are related to the problem(s) rather than to controlling the patient. For example:

> I think, since your heart attack, your heart is under a little strain. You will feel better with some fluid tablets, but you will need some time off work because you will need some time for the heart to recover. I will make you an appointment for some rehabilitation which will help you and get you back to work quicker. Here is a leaflet about what I mean.

This is better than:

> You must stay off work until I tell you. Go for rehabilitation treatment, this will be good for you, and here are some water tablets to take every morning.

Learn to recognise the effect of your own behaviour on your patient. Are you frightening? Do you inspire trust? Do your patients come back to you? What do they tell you about yourself? Learn to recognise, interpret and use your feelings. If you are feeling uneasy and anxious, is your patient feeling that way, too? If you are getting angry, are they, too? Learn to recognise and deal with your own stress. You could read Samuel Shem's *The House of God* (Black Swan Books; 1985). Talk to your friends, and to yourself (but not too much of the latter!). Read the section on 'housekeeping' in *The Inner Consultation*.

With regard to waiting times, most patients don't mind waiting if they are warned that you will be late. Always acknowledge your lateness and make some gesture of apology – hardly anyone will then still object.

Strategies and skills that are helpful when using desktop computers and note-taking

Strategically positioned computer screens should be visible to the patient and a focus for sharing information. A study of MRCGP candidates in 2000 demonstrated that this actually occurs in less than 10% of surgeries. Note-writing and data entry should be kept to a minimum while the patient is present, because they can hinder communication. The truth is that doctors should learn to touch type, as this enables them to record information without losing eye contact with the patient. A useful rule is to read the notes before the consultation and to write them up afterwards. The increasing use of electronic records does allow easier use of the record while one is actually consulting, the quality of the data being the most important factor.

The computer is only a tool – do not let it dictate the agenda (but it does). Read coding (and soon the next type of codes), now essential to modern medical data recording, constrains and limits the boundaries of the consultation. It also tends to emphasise the biomedical model of disease at the expense of the more realistic social and emotional basis of most medical encounters. Computers and their software pose a great threat to the 'art' of medicine, and we as a profession need to devise ways of redressing the balance very soon.

It is sad but true that many patients will take advice from the computer screen more avidly than they will take it from you. Learn to share understanding and clarify the story by using and discussing the information on the screen together. Never enter in the patient's notes or the computer record anything you would not wish your patient to see. Remember that patients have the right of access to their notes and any data about them that are held on computer. All computer systems have the facility to record sensitive information (e.g. previous termination) in such a way as not to be displayed on general view (e.g. to the dismay of the new boyfriend).

Children and their parents

You will quickly learn that children from as young as three are capable of quite complex thought and communication. Many children are more on the ball than their parents. In the surgery they will usually defer to their parents, but this does not mean that they are not listening and understanding. Always take the child into account when giving any explanation, and watch their reaction as well as that of the parent.

It is essential to realise that parents are programmed to worry about their children. They usually fear the worst and are suspicious of doctors underestimating the severity of the illness. Doctors can easily misinterpret this as over-concern or neurosis. For example, consider the scenario of a young mother with a six-month-old baby with some mild vomiting and diarrhoea, already settling by the time she sees you. You believe, with considerable justification, that this is a common, non-worrying and self-limiting condition. However, the mother believes that her baby could be very ill, and specifically that her vomiting could induce a ruptured blood vessel in the stomach and that she could bleed to death – a belief she has acquired from watching a recent soap on television. After the initial exchange and examination, which reveal that the baby is neither ill nor dehydrated, she has only vomited twice and the stools are loose but not watery, the exchange goes something like this:

> Mother: I am very worried about her vomiting.
> Doctor: Don't worry, she isn't dehydrated. Her nappies are still wet, aren't they?
> Mother: Yes, but . . .
> Doctor: Well, I wouldn't worry – give me a ring if she is not settling or her nappies dry out, OK?
> Mother: But the vomiting, doctor?
> Doctor: She is OK, honestly.
> Mother: But are you sure? She is so little.
> Doctor: Yes, of course I am sure. Don't worry, I have seen lots of babies.
> Mother: (increasingly distressed) But could she die, doctor?
> Doctor: (increasingly frustrated) She is not dehydrated, she will be fine. You must not get yourself so worked up.
> Mother: (in tears) I suppose you are right, doctor.

She leaves hurriedly. You are bewildered and think she is anxious and difficult. You make some remark to your partner about young Mrs M being in a right state about a perfectly healthy baby, and blame it on the lack of family support. This is a truly dysfunctional consultation. How might you have prevented it?

You could have avoided this situation by seeking out her concerns. We must always seek out parents' concerns. They may be bizarre, and as we usually couldn't guess them we must ask. In the above example you could have said 'You look really worried. What is it you are frightened of?' The mother might then have told you.

Parents need help to understand their children's illnesses and to get the right perspective. This means that we have to explain clearly, and to give and share information which needs to be consistent with the parents' concerns, beliefs and expressed needs. Special skills are needed for gaining the confidence of children, and these vary with age, sex and temperament. Try to learn from colleagues who have such skills, as there is an art to winning a child's confidence and then persuading them to talk openly to you. As a rough rule of thumb, children respond surprisingly well to being treated in an adult manner, and after the initial surprise they enjoy being involved in the conversation.

The two- or three-way consultations impose a greater strain on our communication skills (e.g. the weeping mum whose two toddlers are spraying ethyl chloride on the new baby's nose and rummaging about in a sharps box which should have been removed weeks ago, while simultaneously screaming that they must go to the loo now). I have no easy solutions for this all too familiar scenario, and would welcome suggestions. What I have learned is to try and put every-thing out of reach of children, but somehow this never works. I always try to stare doe-eyed into the collapsing patient's eyes, and touch her arm to show the required amount of empathy, while inwardly screaming for an electrified crèche several miles away. Sometimes the temptation to chastise the little darlings verbally or physically is almost overwhelming, but it doesn't help the mother. Calm support for her, if possible bolstering her own parental author-ity, is really the order of the day. Reception staff with black belts in judo can sometimes be cajoled into looking after the children for long enough for the mother to get the prescription for Prozac, but the only way to help her properly is either to try to find another time when the kids can be left somewhere else, or to visit her at home and risk that rising-damp feeling as you sink into the sofa just vacated by the nappy-less Tarquin.

Cross-cultural issues

These skills are difficult to acquire and are really beyond the scope of this book, but many regions are experiencing a large increase in the number of such consultations. I must confess to a lack of expertise in this area, but a few strategies come to mind. The first relates to the use of translators. A third party will lengthen the consultation, so you will need more time (often much easier said than done), but more subtly you must be aware that your patient may omit important parts of the history because of embarrassment or worries about confidentiality. If the translator is related to the patient, family dynamics come into play. With all of these variables it can be rather like consulting while wearing a motorcycle helmet with a dirty visor. Signals that you are used to may not mean the same thing, eye contact may be abhorred, a nod may not indicate acceptance, and so on, so your only resort is to keep checking your patient's understanding as best you can. There are now several good texts on this subject, and you should read at least one of them.

Use of the telephone

The telephone is now ubiquitous. In some surgeries more consultations are conducted by telephone than face to face. This form of communication is more difficult, and there are fewer cues, but all the basic rules apply. As the assessment is based solely on the history, and the management plan cannot be reinforced with non-verbal cues, it is especially important to be systematic in covering all of the issues. It has been suggested that training in telephone consultation skills should focus on the following:

- active listening and detailed history taking
- frequent clarification and paraphrasing (to ensure that the messages have been conveyed in both directions)
- picking up cues (e.g. pace, pauses, change in voice intonation)
- providing opportunities to ask questions
- offering patient education
- sharing understanding
- sharing decisions
- arranging appropriate review
- documentation.

When are consultations most likely to go wrong?

1 When we are rushed.
2 When we are interrupted.
3 When we get the wrong notes to start with.
4 When more than one patient consults at once (e.g. mother and children, or husband and wife).

5 When the patient is angry (and when we are angry).
6 When we have a difficult patient.
7 When the patient was expecting to see a different doctor.
8 During evening surgeries! One study found that consultations are three times more likely to go wrong than those in morning surgeries.
9 When the relationship is difficult.
10 When there are real communication problems (e.g. language, speech, idiom, etc.).
11 *Most important of all*, when we don't find out why our patient has really come to see us and what it was that mattered to them.

Chapter 11

Wider communication and ethical issues

'Whole patient medicine'

At its most basic, the concept of 'whole patient medicine' requires doctors to think of other illness, such as a sore throat in a diabetic patient, or a patient presenting with a red eye but who is also severely crippled by arthritis. These descriptions are already clearly reductionist – a characteristic of Western medicine. The more embracing or holistic concepts of the ill person are more usually associated with Eastern thought, or in current Western society with the practitioners of fringe medicine. That this is an ethical issue relates to the effect on the individual. Reductionism and disease orientation encourage the development of teaching such as 'Go and see the liver failure in bed seven and tell me what clinical signs you detect.' There is an inherent conflict between the disease-based medical model and the more socio/psychological models that emphasise unwellness or maladaption of a person in the context of their family and society. Avoiding the worst excesses of this conflict requires doctors to make an effort to see their patients as individuals and, particularly in primary care, to consider the whole person and their medical problems in an embracing rather than exclusive style. This is more difficult for the specialist, and is an ethical reason for regretting the demise of the generalist in hospitals.

Shared decision making and informed consent

The current enthusiasm for shared decision making is a logical development of the earlier concept of informed consent, itself a relatively new and transatlantic concept, having been first mentioned in a Californian supreme court in 1957. There is no doubt that in our present society the idea of informed consent remains very important, very necessary and relates fundamentally to the ability of the medical profession to communicate well with patients. A brief consideration of the history of communication in medicine will indicate what new ideas these are.

The most influential figure in shaping the relationship between doctor and patient over the last 3000 years has probably been Hippocrates. His famous but rather weird oath makes no reference at all to a doctor's duty to converse with patients. In fact, in *Decorum* he admonishes doctors to 'perform their duties calmly and adroitly, concealing most things from the patient . . . revealing nothing of the patient's future or present condition.' Plato, in several of his writings, stated quite categorically that doctors had a right to employ lies for good and noble purposes. This Greek ethic was entrenched in the best of motives – it was thought to be necessary, as the belief was that without respect for medical authority there could be no cure. The idea of the patient participating in decision making was seen as counter-productive. The doctor knew what was best for the patient. The main tenets of Greco-Roman medicine were that patients must honour doctors, for the latter received their authority from God. Patients must therefore have faith in their doctors and must promise obedience. After being around for so long, such ideas do not disappear quickly. How many doctors do you know who still hold views like this?

In the eighteenth and nineteenth centuries a few isolated luminaries suggested educating and involving patients. John Gregory, Professor of Medicine at Edinburgh, was a notable example, and Benjamin Rush, a famous American contemporary of Gregory's, held similar views but, like Gregory, favoured deception whenever enlightenment was not equal to the task. They were both essentially pragmatists, seeking the most effective doctor–patient relationship for therapeutic ends, and not so very concerned about educating patients to share the burdens of decision making.

Some patients were beginning to get a little restless by the middle of the nineteenth century. John Stuart Mill, the famous libertarian, put it quite succinctly in 1859: 'Over himself, his own body and mind, the individual is sovereign.' It took another 100 years for this idea to permeate through to a significant number of the medical profession.

Today the informed consent industry is a growth area, but the product is often rather shoddy. Many doctors still think that telling patients too much is bad for them, despite the existence of overwhelming evidence to the contrary. In fact, patients actually become less anxious if they are adequately informed about major surgical procedures, nasty invasive tests, unpleasant treatments and dangerous drugs.

The American researchers, Greenfield and Kaplan, turned this conundrum on its head. They asked themselves the following question. If doctors do not inform patients too well, what will happen if we teach patients to ask searching questions of their doctors and to negotiate decisions relating to their own care? They took three groups of patients from a Californian hospital – people with peptic ulcers, people with high blood pressure and people with diabetes – and using a randomised technique, they split each group into two, and trained one group to ask appropriate questions and negotiate decisions. They then measured outcomes. So what happened? Lo and behold, in the experimental groups the blood sugar level improved significantly, the blood pressure dropped significantly, ulcers improved more quickly and the patients were happier and liked the involvement. If these results had been achieved by a new diabetic agent – a new ololol or new itidine – the pharmaceutical companies would be ecstatic, but all that was in fact needed was some additional two-way communication.

In 1994, when this book was first published, the anaesthetic department at the Freeman Hospital in Newcastle-upon-Tyne set up a project on postoperative pain relief and the use of self-administering injection pumps. In summary, the patients were using the pumps but were provided with little information and experienced only limited pain relief, although marginally better than that obtained with conventional drug administration. Those patients who received information and explanations from the staff were then given total control of the injection pump containing opiate, etc., and reported dramatic and near total relief of pain. Again a dose of communication gave patients control over their own suffering, with gratifying results.

The fact that informed consent and shared decision making are now such major issues is good for patients, as they are offered more information than ever before. Surgeries overflow with leaflets on every conceivable subject, hospital outpatient departments have printed sheets on most known diseases and procedures, bookshops have huge sections on health and illness, and magazines, radio phone-ins, television programmes and telephone helplines all devote an ever increasing amount of coverage to health-related matters. CD-ROM, DVD and the Internet are now here to stay. While rewriting this chapter I used an Internet search engine to look for references on communication-related matters – there were over 100,000 entries. As early as 1996 a patient of mine with chronic pancreatitis came to me with a sheaf of printouts from Medline asking me to refer him to Dundee, as he had just read their paper on stenting the duct. Whether doctors like it or not, their patients are becoming more informed, and this behaviour is snowballing. There is a change in society's attitude. Although individually patients still tend to adopt a passive role, society as a whole expects the medical profession to educate, inform and involve. The well-known journalist John Illman has produced a booklet for the Association of the British Pharmaceutical Industry (ABPI) entitled *The Expert Patient* (published in 2000), in which he lists a nine-point patient's code. A slightly shortened version is given here.

1 Prepare for the consultation. Write down your symptoms and worries and take the list with you.
2 Be honest, but don't leave things to chance in the hope that they will suddenly disappear. Delay can be dangerous.
3 Be polite. Doctors are not Superman and Superwoman, but ordinary people trying to do a good job. Just like everyone else, they feel more inclined to make an effort for people who show appreciation.
4 Respect your doctor. No one likes to be told how to do their job. An increasing number of patients are demanding treatment from doctors on the basis of information from the Internet or the mass media. By all means discuss any information you have gathered, but ask your doctor which treatment he or she would want in your circumstances.

5 Listen carefully. Take written notes or, even better – if your doctor does not mind – tape-record the consultation.
6 Don't be afraid to ask questions. You may help your doctor to improve his or her communication skills by asking questions if you don't understand the information.
7 Ask about groups that know about your condition. Ask your doctor for details of relevant support groups.
8 Don't be afraid to ask for a second opinion, but be polite about it.
9 Don't be afraid to complain. Again, this is your right, but be polite. Most complaints against doctors are about rudeness and poor communication.

The right to be heard implies the time to be heard. This is a stark fact – many patients find the constraints of short appointments, rushed outpatient appointments, etc., irksome and frustrating. There is evidence that patients make very accurate assessments of how much time they will need with doctors in a primary care setting, as of course they are aware of their own agenda. When patients have been allowed to choose short, medium or long appointments, on the whole this has increased satisfaction for both parties. In ideal well-financed medical systems time is not a problem. It is a further reason why many patients attend fringe medical practitioners. They have bought the time.

Most patients in the UK and the USA are unused to overt rationing, but in the UK covert rationing is the norm, as the demise of the NHS and the rise in managed care have imposed the harsh reality on all. Consumerism, choice, autonomy and rationing produce dissatisfaction and conflict with the medical profession.

True consent is increasingly regarded as a right, and if this right is seen to be denied or infringed, litigation ensues more and more frequently. UK law is still somewhat unclear, but the Sidaway case in England and the Moyes case in Scotland are the most commonly cited precedents. The law does not yet seem to require that fully informed consent should be obtained in all cases, but it does require that important material risks should be disclosed and that all of the patient's questions are answered truthfully. As a criterion for what constitutes a material risk, the 'Bolam' principle applies which, put simply, states that a doctor should act 'in accordance with a practice accepted as proper by a body of responsible and skilled medical opinion' (Lord Diplock). Lord Templeman has emphasised that the amount of medical information that is offered to patients cannot be consistent:

> A patient may make an unbalanced judgement because he is deprived of information. A patient may also make an unbalanced judgement if he is provided with too much information and is made aware of possibilities which he is not capable of assessing because of his lack of medical training, his prejudices, or his personality.

The impact of the new European legislation on human rights has yet to be tested. There has been a seismic shift in attitude and opinion since the 'Bristol case', in which two cardiac surgeons were vilified and humiliated. Although this was partly on account of their poor surgical performance in certain difficult operations on small children, the main complaint by parents concerned the lack of openness and honesty about the chances of success. The expectations of the public with regard to truthful communication by doctors about treatment risks and benefits have never been higher. The discomforting fact for doctors is that much of the information on success rates which was kept from the Bristol parents still remains hidden in many units up and down the UK.

These awful experiences highlight the fact that achieving true informed consent is fraught with difficulties. Most consent is a long way from being informed. Most leaflets are not very good, some are very poor, and some make no sense at all. A northern hospital produced a detailed leaflet on barium studies a few years ago that contained every known risk and complication, and details of preparation. However, it was soon noticed that patients still asked all the old questions. A journalist who was given one of these leaflets had a readability score calculated for it, and discovered that only the most intelligent 1% of the population could understand it. The moral here is that useful information presented in an inaccessible way is useless information. More recently, another northern hospital looked at consent forms for cataract patients and discovered that the print was so small that more than a third of the patients could not read the forms.

A standard hospital technique for obtaining informed consent is to throw information at the patient. The problem is that the information is standardised and the patient is unique – the information will mean different things to different patients depending on their health understanding, and what is readily understandable to one will be incomprehensible to another. A signature of consent may just mean that the patient trusts the doctors, not that they genuinely understand what is to be done to them and what risks there may be. Clinical trials are a really worrying area in this context, as patients tend to assume that any research that they enter into is safe, and American research by the Hastings Center has shown that they do not read consent forms carefully because they assume that someone else has scrutinised the risks and benefits on their behalf. The main motive for enrolling was the belief that the experimental intervention was better than any existing alternative, and that it offered some personal benefit. Doctors' recommendations were, unsurprisingly, found to be very powerful factors influencing the decision to participate in trials. Many of the patients who were interviewed said that they had decided to take part before being given the consent form, and had then not bothered to read it. Doctors are still very influential people, and we must use this influence with care. I have previously mentioned my considerable dislike of the new verb 'to consent' – I sincerely hope that this communication strategy withers on the vine.

It may be that informed consent is already an outmoded concept, and that instead patients should be encouraged to actively request a particular form of treatment after having been adequately informed of the options. This request shifts the onus on to the patient – the consumers of healthcare take responsibility for their choice. This is already happening in some settings, and the Government's patient choice initiative is fuelling the fire. This behaviour was unheard of when I wrote the first edition of this book in 1994. The availability of information from sources such as the Internet is speeding up this transition – our role as doctor is changing from informer to interpreter, so we need to get used to it. The future is now.

In many areas of healthcare, consent is taken for granted because the obvious benefit of the intervention obviates the necessity for any dialogue. Much of the screening/prevention industry works on this premise. In fact, it is often nothing more than a cycle of deceit and half-truths – consent is fudged because true understanding is not easy even for doctors, let alone patients. For example, consider regular breast self-examination, and start with the patient's point of view:

> Regular examination of my own breasts is a good idea because it will stop me from dying of breast cancer.

Well, the bad news is that it won't, or not on present evidence.

> If I find a lump it will mean I will stay healthy because I will have caught it in time.

This is not true, or if it is the difference is not great – operating on some lumps very early may even make the prognosis worse. Some lumps metastasise early and some don't – at present we cannot tell the difference.

> This must be a useful thing to do because the doctor/nurse/ magazine told me to do it.

Really? The Chief Medical Officer did change his mind some years ago, but was howled down and succumbed to encouraging breast awareness, whatever that is, instead.

> It stands to reason it must be a good idea.

It doesn't.

> It makes me worry about cancer, but prevention is better than cure, isn't it?

Not when the premise is a fallacy.
    Now try it from the doctor's point of view.

> It stands to reason it must be a good idea.

Have you looked long and hard at Wilson's criteria for screening recently?

> It cannot do any harm.

It can, not least in creating false expectations and contributing to the overvaluing of medical competence.

> I can't really tell her the truth – she wouldn't believe me.

It would take time, but she might. Honesty should be the best policy.

> But she will think I am an uncaring nihilist and that it does not worry me what happens to her.

If that is the case, you have not achieved any degree of shared understanding and it is still not worth perpetuating a dubious quarter-truth.

Try this exercise with cervical screening, cholesterol measurement, routine private medical screening, mammography, routine colonoscopies, screening for prostate cancer, etc., and ask yourself how much of the consent is really informed. There is a major ethical divide between your patient coming to you for your opinion and help with their agenda, and you imposing your screening agenda on that patient. If you do initiate such a procedure, you should have conclusive evidence that the test is likely to alter the outlook for that individual favourably, and that it is most unlikely to do any physical or psychological harm. You must face the issues honestly and help your patient to ask searching questions. At last the main body of the medical profession is waking up to this shameful state of affairs. The *British Medical Journal* produced a landmark edition in September 1999, entitled *Embracing Patient Partnership* (it has a picture of a couple dancing the tango on the front cover). A leading article by Joan Austoker attacks the screening industry, and her final paragraph is worth quoting in full:

> Nevertheless, although uncertainties complicate the process of achieving informed consent, they underscore the importance of conducting research and taking care to ascertain what people believe about the disease and its causes, what they understand, and what they want to know. Ultimately informed patient choice, particularly about interventions that are both offered and delivered by health professionals, should take place in the context of shared decision making between the patient and health professional. Above all, we need to respect patients' autonomy – and that includes their right to decide not to undergo a screening intervention, even when refusal may result in harm to themselves.

The issue of screening for most patients is often that it is a necessary evil that is likely to confer health benefits. The possibility that screening may have harmful or negative effects is not often considered, but when faced by doctors communicating the results of screening there is much greater scepticism. In a study conducted in Australia, women patients carefully watched their doctor's non-verbal behaviour when they were receiving the results of their pap smear, in order to reach a conclusion about the doctor's veracity. The underlying issue was that of not trusting physicians to tell the whole truth.

In order to obtain true informed consent for cervical screening, doctors should:

- inform women of the limitations and disadvantages of the test
- inform women that the absolute benefit, to them as individuals, of their participation in the screening programme is extremely small
- inform women that as such screening accounts for part of the general practitioner's income, there may be a conflict of interest
- check to ensure that women understand the issues
- read the General Medical Council's booklet, *Seeking Patients' Consent: the ethical considerations*.

The ethics of the doctor's agenda

This is a complex area that has received too little attention in the past. Again it relates to the implicit contract between doctor and patient, and the difficulties are most easily highlighted by a discussion of lifestyle advice and screening. Many doctors believe that the right to give unsolicited health and lifestyle advice is inherent in the nature of the relationship. The principle of beneficence comes into play – if the advice is for the patient's good it is ethically justified. Doctors who adhere strongly to such beliefs will view it as unethical to withhold such advice. Not all doctors would agree with this, and many find this a grey area, some developing an internalised scale of intrusiveness versus perceived benefit to the patient's health future. Some physicians who place patient autonomy high on their list of priorities will seldom offer such advice. Several authors, such as Illich, Skrabanek, McCormick and Iona Heath in her Pickles Lecture of 1999, have warned against any further unsolicited encroachments of medical advice into society, arguing about the dangers, the fallacies and the inherent uncertainty of widespread interference by doctors in the everyday lives of people in society.

To quote Heath, an eminent GP working in Kentish Town, London:

> Medical science has valued the simple statistics of longevity above any measures of the quality of life. Many of our patients' palpable lack of enthusiasm for the 'lifestyle advice' we are obliged to deliver tells a different story, but the reordering of priorities is nonetheless both insidious and pernicious . . . Much more work needs to be done to analyse and describe the limitations of biomedical science, the importance of death, and the overwhelming need to incorporate the patients' own values and aspirations into a system of care which is increasingly driven by standardised protocols. We must recognise the tendency for medical science to become totalitarian.

The insidious nature of this advice has been described as *coercive healthism*. The medical profession can easily slip into the role of the main arbiter of what is good for people, creating a climate of unjustified fear in an otherwise extremely healthy society. This whole (probably unstoppable) development is a major barrier to personal autonomy and a continuation of the old beneficent paternalism, and there is a further danger of the doctor making negative value judgements when a conflict of health interests arises. A blaming culture arises, especially when doctors perceive that the patients could do more to help themselves. Smoking and obesity often arouse strong victim-blaming reactions in doctors, producing unempathetic and often rather abrupt communication styles. The widespread rise in alcoholism and drug abuse has fuelled this difficulty, with many doctors stating that they will not treat such individuals. The spread of AIDS has in some cases brought the worst out of the medical profession (as well as the best). These behaviours in patients pose severe ethical problems for caring doctors – more so in organisations such as the NHS and managed care, where resources are clearly finite. Achieving a balance between beneficence, autonomy and justice is difficult. The communication imperative for the doctor should still be one of understanding and developing the autonomy of the individual. Issues of fairness, rationing and justice are better left outside the consulting-room if at all possible.

The rise of the screening industry highlights this dilemma further. Health is seen as a commodity, immediately turning patients into consumers and consigning doctors to the role of middle managers in a health industry. New words are used. Old-style doctoring is replaced by 'anticipatory care', 'prevention' (which in this context only means a promise of a decreased likelihood of an event) and the now ubiquitous 'proactive.' As in Orwell's *1984*, language is used to conceal truth. The ethics of the relationship change dramatically. With good information the patient can decide on the risks and benefits of the procedure. If handled properly, this can lead to acceptable informed consent and an ethically defensible contract, but as already stated many of the existing screening programmes short-circuit the consent issue. Some are even deliberately economical with the truth, emphasising the benefits while playing down the uncertainties, risks and detrimental effects. Again, apologists will cite the beneficent arguments while playing down autonomy.

Western societies are increasingly concerned about health, paradoxically at a time when it has never been better. Individual patients vary with regard to their own personal concern. Some people have always had an unhealthy obsession with health, as Mark Twain pointed out:

> There are people who strictly deprive themselves of each and every eatable, drinkable and smokeable which has in any way acquired a shady reputation. They pay this price for health. And health is all they get out of it. It is like paying out your whole fortune for a cow that has gone dry.

Patients for whom personal health, prevention, well-being and longevity are high on their agenda are also invoking their right to be heard. This can pose problems in predominantly disease- and problem-based systems of care. Conflicts of agenda can arise, autonomy coming into conflict with justice in the form of time rationing. The place of these issues in the primary care consultation remains unresolved.

One of our difficulties in the new millennium is that our agenda as doctors is being constantly expanded, with uncertain consequences for patients. The cholesterol debate illustrates this increasing nightmare. As I write it is now agreed that secondary prevention of heart disease by lowering cholesterol is a good and evidence-based strategy for our population. This means that all patients with any suggestion of heart trouble come under the umbrella of medical care for the rest of their lives. Fair enough, I hear you say, and you might be right. The next step, suggested by trials on high-risk but healthy men in the West of Scotland, is that most of us should take cholesterol-lowering drugs for the rest of our lives. Apart from the horrendous cost to the Exchequer, this means that most of the adult population will become patients. We are now bombarded by frightening-looking journals full of statistics about the numbers of people who need to be treated for so many years in order to prevent some event. I still do not know how this really helps me to treat worried Mr Hay sitting next to me. I do know that we are both going to die of something, and that my job as his doctor is to help him to live as healthy a life as possible in the context of our society. We shall all need to be informed on this debate, have our cholesterol monitored and increase the burden on the health industry. It seems that Ivan Illich is right, and that we are increasingly medicalising all aspects of our lives. This worries me. Does it worry you?

Hypertension – as I said in Chapter 5, a doctor's disease if ever there was one – has now reached plague proportions. Depending on which set of guidelines you use, over 50% of over-75s should be on active treatment. If you stand back from this thought for a second, you begin to wonder if the lunatics are taking over the asylum. Let me remind you that this is not a benign diagnosis. Irrespective of treatment, the diagnosis is associated with an 80% increase in absenteeism, sport is avoided, impotence rates quadruple, and the 'hypertensive' person now sees him- or herself differently. They become preoccupied with sickness and their energy levels decline. In one study using the Quality of Life Impairment Scale, 30% of patients classified them-selves as 'severely ill.' This is a label that makes people sick, so we doctors have to do an awful lot of good to make up for it. David Misselbrook, in his excellent book *Thinking About Patients*, suggests that you ask all of your hypertensive patients three questions:

1 Do you ever wonder if you might be experiencing side-effects from your medication?

2   Do you often think about your blood pressure?
3   Does your blood pressure cause you any problems in your day-to-day life?

He found very high levels of anxiety and a feeling of being stigmatised by the label. Try it yourself.

The real crux of the whole informed consent debate is that to obtain true informed consent requires the achievement of *a shared understanding and a shared management plan.* This further implies that the patient's beliefs should be known and their understanding checked effectively. The ethical imperative behind achieving a shared understanding is respect for the individual. To achieve these tasks at all requires a belief by the physician that sharing with patients is a desirable outcome. This is not and never can be a framework for paternalistic consulting. Ethically this has to be a true belief, not a Machiavellian means of achieving the outcome desired by the doctor. Most doctors are not that pure and, while espousing the patient-centred method, will use it to manipulate the patient in a beneficent but paternalistic way. There is an assumption that consent can never be truly informed, so that it is for doctors to determine what is in the patient's best interest. However, health is mainly the subjective experience of an individual and is made up of highly personal beliefs, feelings and experiences. It follows that, when helped by physicians to achieve a comprehension of the risks and benefits of various treatments, it is patients and only patients who can really determine which therapy will help them to achieve their most important health goals.

It has always seemed to me that one of the ethical hallmarks of good consulting is a requirement for honesty. There is an imperative for the doctor to seek and confirm understanding in four main areas: first, that the patient is aware that they are an active part of the decision-making process; secondly, that they are aware of the choices; thirdly, that they are aware of the implications of those choices; and finally that they have assimilated enough specific information on the risks and benefits to allow them to make an informed choice. Sadly, although this may be the ideal ethical position, recordings of consultations of young GPs suggest that such behaviour is by no means the norm.

The communication of risk–benefit advice is an interesting area. This is communication at its most difficult, and in this age of evidence-based choice doctors will need to learn to do it well. Patients who are well informed will often make choices of which doctors may not approve. The medical benefits of stroke prevention by warfarin in atrial fibrillation seem to be clear, but in a group of patients who were well informed of the risks and benefits, a significant proportion decided not to choose the intervention. Several studies have demonstrated that the method of communicating risk significantly affects patient uptake. Numbers needed to treat patients with mild hypertension in order to prevent one event provide a very different perspective to saying that taking a particular intervention halves an already small risk. This is an area where 'framing' the questions can easily distort the truth, whatever that is – 'spin' is a more popular word for the same idea. For example, most doctors are likely to tell patients that trials show that treatment is indicated for mild hypertension, and that treatment will prevent them from having a stroke. They won't usually say that there is a 99.8% probability that treatment will do the individual no good in any given year, that treatment fails to prevent the majority of strokes, and that the very marginal benefits of treatment need to be set against the anxiety, medicalisation, side-effects and expense of treatment. The scope for unethical and manipulative behaviour is very wide, often fuelled by the profit-related motives of pharmaceutical companies.

The major problem with risk is the differing frames of reference used by patients and doctors. Doctors use mathematical concepts, absolute risk, relative risk and numbers needed to treat. Patients with varying loci of control see themselves, for very unmathematical reasons, as being high, medium or low risk, and then use the lottery logic of luck, fate and destiny to make an individual and unique assessment. If we let them, our patients will tell us compelling stories to communicate their perceptions to us, having already swapped stories in the pub in order to construct their own sense of reality. We doctors, on the other hand, relate statistics but without the persuasive reality and impact of the stories our patients relate. It means that doctors could do worse than learn to relate counter-stories to combat our patients' tales – this is high-level communication and is likely to be unusual. The burning unanswerable question our patient wants to ask is 'Do you really think that taking this tablet for the next 30 years is definitely going to do me more good than harm?' I don't know if you back horses, but most gamblers wouldn't touch the odds for 'treating' mild hypertension. Interestingly, numbers needed to treat (NNTs) are quite difficult to find at present, but the *Bandolier* website is your best bet. You could also try the website of the Oxford Centre for Evidence-Based Medicine. You should also read an article entitled 'Communicating risks: illusion or truth?', published in the *British Medical Journal* in September 2003.

Patient utilities is an expression that has been gaining ground since the earlier editions of this book. It is a rather inelegant American way of defining what matters to patients. This has allowed us to rethink some older but interesting measures, such as von Neumann's 'Standard Gamble', which balances the negative utility of a particular outcome against a risk of sudden death, and tries to define what risk an individual is actually prepared to take. Another is Torrance's 'Time Trade-Off', which defines the value of improvements in health by a comparison with the life expectancy that an individual is prepared to forgo in order to achieve them. Misselbrook again advocates a new measure, which is the inverse of NNTs, that he calls the 'Personal Probability of Benefit' (PPB), and he goes on to argue that if we do not explain the low probability of benefit to patients there can be no informed consent.

When trying to achieve shared decision making, it is permissible – perhaps even morally obligatory – for a doctor to attempt by negotiation to change the mind of a patient who is making an apparently silly or irrational choice. It is through these genuine negotiations that the doctor and patient can come to a truly shared understanding of the issues in a way that is best suited to maximising the values of both. However, although the decision-making process is shared, the final decision is that of the patient. It has to be said though that it must be correct, in extreme cases of conflict of belief, for physicians to retain the power not to treat patients if the management choice and plan require them to act in a manner that they believe is unethical.

A good model must be one of *mutual persuasion* by two experts, one on medical matters and the other on their own mind and body. This implies that doctors must be prepared to allow themselves to be persuaded by their patients away from their first or second choices of action if the patient's argument is effective, convincing and – most importantly – informed. Doctors are not always going to like this.

Any general practitioner who wants to be an effective doctor must be interested in people and not merely diseases. They must be committed to their patients' welfare, willing to search out their patients' beliefs, and it follows that they must also be willing to listen to whatever problems the patients bring to them. This is an intensely personal form of doctoring, which is not seen in hospitals very often. The treatment of a disease can be largely impersonal, but the care of a patient is entirely personal.

The General Medical Council is unequivocal in its position on the duties of a doctor:

> Patients must be able to trust doctors with their lives and well-being. To justify that trust, we as a profession have a duty to maintain a good standard of practice and care and to show respect for human life. In particular, as a doctor you must:
>
> - make the care of your patient your first concern
> - treat every patient politely and considerately
> - respect patients' dignity and privacy
> - listen to patients and respect their views
> - give patients information in a form that they can under-stand
> - respect the right of patients to be fully involved in decisions about their care
> - keep your professional knowledge and skills up to date
> - recognise the limits of your professional competence
> - be honest and trustworthy
> - respect and protect confidential information
> - make sure that your personal beliefs do not prejudice your patients' care
> - act quickly to protect patients from risk if you have good reason to believe that you or a colleague may not be fit to practise
> - avoid abusing your position as a doctor
> - work with colleagues in the ways that best serve patients' interests.

In all of these matters you must never discriminate unfairly against your patients or colleagues. And you must always be prepared to justify your actions to them.

(*Source:* General Medical Council. *Duties of a Doctor.* London: General Medical Council; 2000)

Chapter 12

Special situations and patients

Breaking bad news

This is not easy to do, and it can be such a daunting prospect that many doctors try all sorts of diversions and strategies to avoid doing it. 'Nurses are so much better at that sort of thing' is often the excuse given. The reasons for this shying away from the task are probably primarily emotional. Causing distress in another person causes distress in us. Therefore many of us do not perform very well in this crucial area of doctor–patient communication.

Common faults when breaking bad news

- Just not doing it, and hoping that someone else will pick up the pieces, such as the GP, another colleague, one of the nursing staff, etc. Common methods of doing this include avoiding the patient, never seeing them alone, or always being in a hurry.
- Putting off the evil hour.

> I think we should do some more investigations.

- Lying, or at best being 'economical with the truth.'

> We took the whole breast away and the affected glands. I am sure we took it all away.
> You will soon be better after the chemotherapy.
> No, it's not too serious, we can cure it for you.

- Deliberately not picking up patient cues.

> I seem to be fading away, doctor.
> Really? How are you sleeping?
> The treatment isn't working, is it, doctor?
> Well, perhaps you are a little constipated.

- Going into undertaker mode, with excessive solemnity and an aura of deepening gloom. Lying is one thing, but excessive objectivity without mitigation is just as bad.
- Avoiding social and emotional issues. A study of oncologists in 1996 found that the doctors used closed questions and seldom gave the patients space to initiate any discussion. Although the patients must have been frightened, with all sorts of fears, only 1% of their talk was related to their concerns. To use a bit of jargon discussed earlier, the level of 'patient-centredness' was very low. In this study patients were well informed about their diagnosis, prognosis and treatment options, but their emotional well-being was rarely probed. There were almost no social questions from the doctors, and the researchers found that the level of expressed empathy from the doctors was as low as 1%.
- Not recognising that emotion may block the patient's ability to take in much information.

Useful strategies to help you break bad news to patients

- Honesty is the best policy. Never tell patients anything that you know is not true. The truth will emerge over time, and the feelings of betrayal and of being misled will surface and sour your relationship both with your patient and with their family.
- Do not, however, tell the patient more than they want to know. This implies the need for a skilful manoeuvre to find out how much information they can cope with.
- Take great care with prognostications. *Never* give a specific time period – it will only come back to haunt you. You will almost certainly be wrong, and the effect on your patient will be depres-

sing. Hope will ebb away and anxiety will increase as the stated time approaches. However, most patients do want some guidance on what the future holds for them.

- Do not remove all hope. Find some reason to be optimistic. The condition may be terminal, but you can encourage the patient to look forward to a particular event, such as a birth or celebration of an anniversary, or they may be hoping for a period of remission or for a peaceful, pain-free death.
- Remember the duty of confidentiality that is owed to your patient. This tends to go out of the window as soon as serious illness is suspected. Doctors have become used to ushering spouses into darkened corners and whispering terrible intimate details of their loved one's condition without a by-your-leave to the unfortunate sufferer. This has always been assumed to be for the patient's well-being. A study reported in the *British Medical Journal* in 1996 concluded that almost all patients, however ill, wanted to know their diagnosis, and most of them wanted to know about the prognosis, treatment options and side-effects. In the same issue another study showed that patients rejected unconditional dis-closure of information without their consent. They valued respect for their autonomy more highly than the medical beneficence, and considered that their own needs took priority over those of their family.
- Follow-up after giving bad news is especially important.

Useful skills to help you break bad news to patients

- Use your eliciting skills as described in Chapter 10.
- Ask yourself the question 'How might this news affect this patient?' Think of the patient's family setting and their psycho-logical make-up. Many patients are more worried about the effect of the bad news on others than they are about themselves.
- Consider the use of a tape recorder. This technique is now being used with increasing frequency in oncology departments. The evidence suggests that the patients and their relatives listen to the recordings on several occasions.
- Ask patients directly how much they know about the 'bad news.' For example, remember Mrs Arthur. Let us suppose that a thyroid

scan has suggested a malignancy in one of the nodules, and a biopsy has confirmed this. She comes back to you for the report and your advice on further treatment. How do you proceed? Try the following type of approach:

Mrs Arthur: I have been so worried, doctor. What did the biopsy show?

Doctor: Do you know why we did the biopsy?

Mrs Arthur: Yes, to see if it was cancer. Was it that, doctor?

Doctor: Yes, it was. I know that is bad news, but the outlook is not as bad as you think. Tell me what thyroid cancer means to you.

Mrs Arthur: Does this mean it will spread right through me? Will I die?

Doctor: No on both counts. We should be able to remove the gland and the cancer, and make sure it does not return by giving you some radiation treatment.

Mrs Arthur: That doesn't sound very nice – are you sure you can stop the cancer?

Doctor: There is always a risk we can't, but you would be very unlucky. The treatment I mentioned is very effective. Would you like to speak to someone more expert than me about it?

Mrs Arthur: Well, not today, but could I bring my husband along to see you and perhaps the other doctor you just mentioned?

- There is a lot more information you could give Mrs Arthur, and she may well want it, in time, but using the patient-centred approach as above enables the patient to take in only as much information with its unpleasant implications as they can cope with at one sitting.
- Be especially sensitive. Abrupt and brutal honesty, associated with authoritarian patient control, has no place in modern medicine. For example, consider the case of Mrs Arthur again. The following type of approach is not recommended:

> The test shows it's cancer I'm afraid. We are bringing you in tomorrow morning to have the gland out. You can't hang around when cancer is about. OK?

- You must show consideration for your patient's feelings. Allow them time to think of questions and then you must answer them, and assure them of ongoing support. It is much better if bad news is given in the context of a continuing, supportive relationship. Do not give bad news and then make a run for it. Sit down with your patient and take your time. A pleasant, warm and safe setting is preferable. Try to ensure that there is someone else with the patient when you leave. You may need (with the patient's permission) to contact their partner or a close friend.
- When discussing the prognosis, remember that if your patient asks 'How long have I got?', they are already formulating an answer. You could say something like 'Well, I know you are poorly, but I think you have some time left, but how does it look to you?' Their answer may help you to deepen the discussion. What about the question 'Shall I ask my brother to come back from Australia?' I try answering this question with another: 'Well, put yourself in his shoes. How would you feel if you were too late?'
- Learn to recognise and cope with *denial*. We all deal with devastating news in different ways. Many people cope by using varying degrees of denial. During your career you will experience situations where you have what you consider to be a sensitive, honest chat with a patient, containing a great deal of information, and then at the next consultation the patient will completely deny having had the conversation: 'They never told me anything at the hospital.'
- It is not a good strategy to break down denial too brutally. It is there for a purpose. Respect for the individual should extend to their defence mechanisms. This does not mean that we ourselves have to be a party to the denial and start encouraging unrealistic expectations. We must still reply honestly to any questions. It also means that we must pick up on rather obvious patient cues such as 'The hospital doctor said it was just a little tumour. What a relief it isn't cancer, doctor.'

- Family denial or collusion is another problem more commonly encountered in general practice.

> Don't tell him, doctor, it will kill him.

- This can lead to a tragic conspiracy of silence. The sufferer knows full well that their condition is terminal, but they cannot talk to their loved ones for fear of upsetting them. The loved ones in turn are so afraid of upsetting the sufferer in their last few weeks that nothing about the illness, about dying, about saying goodbye, etc., is discussed – to the detriment of all concerned. Spouses collude because they love their other half and they don't want to hurt them – collusion is always a two-way process.
- Here I think there is a place for sensitive intervention by the doctor to try to break this pernicious circle. I believe firmly that our responsibility is to the patient, and that any responsibility to the family is secondary. In this type of situation we should tell the relatives that we would not impose the truth on the patient, but that if the patient asks we shall not lie. Often, with experience and tact, we can persuade all parties to talk reasonably openly about the future and help the patient towards a much more rewarding death, with a normal and not exaggerated grief to follow. This facilitation of family dynamics can be one of the more satisfying events in which we doctors can become involved.
- Use emotive words with care. Whatever the words 'cancer', 'tumour', 'growth', 'metastases', 'vegetative', 'malignant', 'thrombosis', etc., mean to you, it is certain that they do not mean the same thing to your patient. Check their understanding frequently, and remember that some people, cultures and societies have taboos relating to words like cancer. Be careful.
- Give your patient space to take it in. Pause, touch, empathise, commiserate, and use silence. Try to help to pick up the pieces. This can be emotionally painful for you, too.
- Remember that for the patient this is a momentous occasion. People recall the how, where and when very clearly, and you – as the doctor – are wielding immense power. A woman of my

acquaintance told me that when the young hospital doctor gave her better than expected news about her cancer, 'I was so pleased I could have married him.'

- Be prepared to spread the explanations over several consultations. It can help to ask the patient to write down questions as they come into their head and to bring them along to the next consultation.
- It is also true that what is bad news for one person may not be so for another. I was commiserating with an old patient of mine about her dying husband when she exploded: 'Don't worry about me, doc. The old bugger has been driving me mental for years. The quicker he goes the better.'
- Just to recap, a paper published in the *British Medical Journal* in 2004 described a study from Canada and Australia of what patients receiving palliative care for cancer wanted to know. Six doctor attributes necessary for sensitive sharing of information were identified:
  - playing it straight
  - staying the course
  - giving time
  - showing that you care
  - making it clear
  - pacing the information.

Angry patients

This is another difficult emotional area, especially if the anger is directed towards you or one of your colleagues. Being ill can make people angry, so doctors are going to encounter a lot more than their fair share of this emotion. There are many reasons why patients get angry, including excessive waiting times and delayed appointments. Distress for another, often mixed with righteous indignation about the perceived medical failings, sometimes results in very intense and unpleasant encounters. There may be concerns that the patient feels have not been taken seriously, disappointment at the lack of therapeutic success, and simple misunderstandings (especially when the patient expects one treatment but receives another, and the doctor has failed to explain the rationale). Guilt felt by patients or relatives that somehow they should have come sooner or cared for the patient better is a common reason for anger being directed at doctors. Anger is natural in grief and when adjusting to a serious diagnosis – the 'Why me?' effect. For most angry patients and relatives anxiety is often the trigger.

Strategies for recognising and dealing with angry patients

- Remember that it is the patient who is angry, not you. This may be difficult, depending on your temperament. It is all too common for a simple misunderstanding to develop into a huge row, the worst place for this being reception, where other patients can watch and take sides.
- Do not leave the anger unexplored. Glowering at each other throughout the consultation is not effective and is bad for coronary arteries.
- Use your own feelings. If you are feeling angry, it is very likely that the patient is, too. Doctors feel anger if their competence is questioned or if they feel that their integrity is being challenged. After all, doctors are human, too, and a lack of appreciation from palpably ungrateful patients can make us cross, especially if we feel that we have made a special effort.
- Be patient – anger does not usually last for long.
- Always support your staff in the face of aggression that is really aimed at you. This is both a moral suggestion and a practical one. If you don't provide such support, before long you will not have any staff left.

Skills for defusing angry patients

- When you recognise anger, gentle confrontation may be helpful.

> You seem to be cross about something.
> Help, you do look upset.
> Come on, get it off your chest, what is bothering you?
> You were very angry with the nurse/receptionist. Why was that?

- In communication terms anger has a purpose – to gain the listener's (in this case the doctor's) complete attention. It is wise to let this happen.
- When you are listening, maintain non-threatening eye contact. Try not to raise your eyebrows, purse your lips or adopt an aggressive stance. When you speak, break off eye contact from time to time to demonstrate your wish to be conciliatory.
- Deal with the main issue first. Summarise the main points and then check them.
- Acknowledge the frailties and imperfections of medical diagnosis and treatment. Again honesty remains the best policy. A perceived delay in diagnosis or treatment is a common cause of patient anger. However, frankness about the nature of the delay will often defuse this.
- Acknowledge your own lack of omnipotence, and watch the effects of your own guilt feelings. If you do not bring some of these feelings into the open, your relationship may be irrevocably harmed. I visited a little girl some time ago and thought that she had mild flu. A few hours later my partner admitted her with acute lobar pneumonia. The parents were angry about my perceived incompetence and told my partner so, and I was angry with myself and felt guilty for missing the diagnosis. I went to see the family, feeling rather ill at ease, after the little girl had been discharged, and I expressed my pleasure at her recovery and my regrets about not diagnosing the pneumonia. The mother said:

> It was not your fault, doctor. You did examine her and you can't be right all the time. It did come on pretty quickly.

And the family continued to be my patients.

- When there seems to be a real threat of physical violence, and you have made every effort to defuse the situation, avoid physical confrontation. If possible, move away and get help. If you have a panic button, press it.

The somatising patient

Another common difficulty is the patient who attends repeatedly with physical illness that is unclassifiable by an increasingly investigative doctor. The unexplained breathlessness, the flitting chest pains, the weird pins and needles – all possible precursors of nasty diseases. However, we have to remember that common things are common, most illnesses are not serious and most symptoms are not disease. They are problems of living turned into symptoms by anxious people and turned into disease by biologically trained doctors. Patients who are prone to turning inner anxieties into symptoms are called somatisers. Doctors who turn such symptoms into disease have been called medicalisers. As I mentioned in Chapter 5, a medicalising doctor and a somatising patient are a bad combination.

These are the patients we find especially difficult, the ones who ask 'What are you going to do about my (whatever it is)?' They get labelled 'heartsink' patients in general practice, and in hospital they are very quickly 'turfed' from the senior staff to their junior colleagues. The really chronic somatiser does not have their notes inspected – they have them weighed. This sad, irritating and enormously time-consuming state of affairs is the result of a long process of medicalisation by doctors and the health industry, including alternative medicine, of essentially nervous and functional complaints made by introspective individuals. These people often have a 'powerful other' locus of control, although fussy internal controllers can get doctors down. Curiously, fatalists do not commonly produce such negative emotions.

The problem with doctors in this context is that if patients keep pushing we will eventually do something. This could be a test, which will lead to a procedure, which can lead to an operation, which can lead to a complication, which in turn will reinforce the patient's inappropriate health-seeking behaviour.

> See, I was ill, doctor. I am a lot better after my triple artery graft. Now about these headaches . . .

I know personally a group of patients who have had coronary artery surgery – not because their arteries were in any worse shape than most, but because they persistently kept presenting different symptoms to different doctors. This led to tests being performed that were equivocal, as tests tend to be, but the pressure for something to be done meant that in the end something was done. These patients had thick sets of notes before and even thicker ones afterwards. So what can we doctors do about this?

Strategies for decreasing our patients' tendency to become somatically fixated and medically dependent

- Use the communication methods described earlier in this book, with particular emphasis on achieving a shared understanding and shared management plan. Patients should be encouraged to take some responsibility for their own health.
- Use the traditional disease-based medical model with care. Although we all need to be good diagnosticians, good efficient clinical practice demands balances – most headaches do not warrant MRI scans – investigation on demand is bad medicine, and treatment on demand may be worse. We must not create disease where only poor individual coping mechanisms are the problem. This can mean trying to change the patient's purely biomechanical view of illness. Psychologists call this the defusion of the organic versus the functional, and they use strategies to help patients to 'reattribute' their explanations for ill health. These strategies include emphasising the role of anxiety in muscular tension, pain and hyperventilation, the effect of depression on pain thresholds, and the vicious circle of pain and psychological distress.
- Be on your guard against manipulative behaviour, which is a common feature of the somatising patient.
- Avoid referral if at all possible. Only when all reasonable avenues and likely diagnoses have been refuted should a referral be made. I still believe that one of the general practitioner's primary duties is to protect his or her patients from hospital medicine. Hospital medicine is almost exclusively disease-based; patients must be

diagnosed thoroughly and possible causes ruled out. Once an anxious, introspective patient gets to outpatients the die is cast – investigation is coming and all that that might entail. The fixation with the symptom will be intensified and the vicious self-reinforcing loop encouraged. Referrals should only be made for the following reasons:

for *diagnostic reasons* (i.e. the further testing of a specific hypothesis, the resources for which you do not possess)

- for *therapeutic purposes* (if you do not want or are unable to treat a certain condition)
- for *reassurance*. This is the really tricky one. Even if there is no traditional disease, the modern hospital's ability to dig up some minor disorder which is essentially irrelevant, and to over-treat it, is formidable. This can of course lead to further referral. There is also the danger that, not unreasonably, you or your chief may ask the patient to return on the grounds that although you have drawn a blank, you may have overlooked something. Both of these situations will probably lead the patient to conclude that they were right, and that there is something wrong with their health. For example, the 42-year-old woman patient with atypical chest pain who insisted on referral has a non-specific minor anomaly in a couple of leads of the ECG. This leads to echocardiography which is essentially OK, and to a treadmill test which is also essentially OK, but with a performance nearer the bottom end of the normal range than the top. This leads to a full catheterisation, which is essentially normal, but no one's arteries are entirely normal, and the patient overhears your discussion of her essentially normal variants with rising anxiety. Her consequent release of catecholamines and irritation of previously untouched places by the catheter produce a minor arrhythmia that you need to respond to quickly and (in her eyes) dramatically. Her worst fears are confirmed and the seeds of cardiac crippledom are well and truly sown.

- The reasons for referral should be explicit, and the doctor who accepts the referral should whenever possible keep within the mandate of the referral letter.

- Try to keep the numbers of doctors involved with a particular patient to a minimum. The more doctors there are involved, the more somatisation there will be.
- Keep good records. You need to let partners and other doctors know what your plans are, whether you fear a somatising process is happening to the patient and your strategies for preventing further harm.
- Communicate with your colleagues about patients you suspect of undue somatisation leading to 'doctor shopping' (i.e. consulting every doctor in the practice in turn for another opinion, or swapping specialists frequently).
- Write explicit and detailed referral letters. These should contain biographical details, clinical and physical symptoms and signs, the course of the complaint, your own hypotheses, previous history, important psychosocial background, and the beliefs and wishes of the patient. There should also be a clear statement of what you are asking of your colleague, and what you wish to happen after your colleague has seen the patient.
- Use patient diaries and other methods of self-recording to try to produce more insight and linkage between events and symptoms.

Skills for preventing and dealing with somatisation

- Use the concepts of transactional analysis. You are trying to achieve an adult–adult relationship, not a parent–child relationship. Read Eric Berne's *Games People Play*.
- Discuss your perceptions of your patient's illness behaviour.

> You have been coming to see me a lot recently, and I never seem to find much wrong. What do you expect of me?
> It is a year since your heart attack and you still seem to be leaving everything to your wife. It is as if you do not want to get better.

- Discuss the patient's methods of denial and avoidance.

> Every time I ask you if anything is troubling you, you say to me 'nobody has a perfect life' and leave it at that, but you keep coming to me with problems that I can't really help you with. You will have to help me more before I can help you.
>
> I know you have not been well in the last year. Today it is your sinuses, last time it was your tummy pain and before that your headaches. Do you think there is something worrying you underneath all this?
>
> You are trying to blame everything on a virus, but I think you are not facing the real problem of your anxiety.

- Try to verbalise your patient's anxiety.

> You are afraid it is something serious, aren't you?
>
> You seem very tense. Are you frightened of something?
>
> If you go on worrying about yourself you are going to get into a vicious circle, don't you think?
>
> You have been panicking a bit recently, but nothing serious has developed. Can you get any comfort from that?

- Use the presenting signals from the minimal cues.

> You seem much more anxious than normal.
>
> It looks to me that something is really troubling you.

- Describe to the patient the way in which they are trying to influence you.

> I know you would like me to send you to see a specialist, but I do not think that is necessary. I am not sure what to do next.
> I think you want me to give you a pill and then expect all your troubles will be over, but I don't think it is as easy as that.
> The way you are behaving gives me the feeling you are saying 'Please help me, I don't know which way to turn.' Am I right?

- Discuss and use your own feelings.

> Honestly I have tried everything and I don't know where to go from here. Have you any suggestions?
> I am sorry, but you have made me feel inadequate and unable to help you. Can you help me to help you?

- Clarify the patient's complaint(s), to give them more insight.

> I think your headache is caused by the muscles in the neck going into spasm. This is why painkillers don't work very well – they don't relieve the spasm. It is probably your worrying about your Mum that caused the muscle spasm in the first place.

- Try to avoid giving too much advice to these patients. Any advice should be specific (i.e. to give a new approach to the problem), and it should be realistically tailored to the individual patient.
- Encourage the patient's internal search, and encourage them to find their own solutions and alternative strategies.
- Don't let such patients get you down.

Remember that many patients with somatising disorders are depressed as well as anxious.

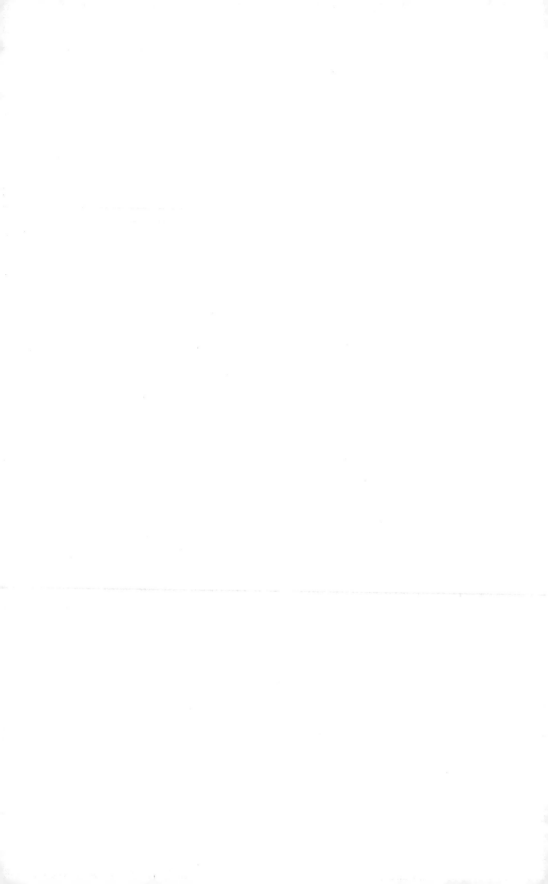

Chapter 13

Summary

I wonder what you have learned from this book? The message I hope you will take away is that effective communication can be learned. That it is not just God-given and incapable of improvement. We can all do it better, but we have to believe that the effort is worthwhile and that the goal is an important one.

Let me summarise some of the very important messages, firstly about patients.

What doctors should know about patients

In hospital

The patient is more frightened than you are. They think that their condition is more serious than you do. Most of them want to be involved in their own treatment, and want to understand what is going to happen to them.

They have not come to you about liver or thyroid disease. They have come because of their beliefs about, their expectations of and the effects of their perceived change in health. Remember, whenever possible, to try to put yourself in their shoes.

Your patient is probably afraid of you. They will tend to be passive and not say very much. This does not mean that they do not want to know.

Patients are just people like you. They deserve respect, they need to be informed and they need to consent. However, people are all different, they respond to a change in health in different ways and they need individual, personalised plans.

People can easily have inappropriate and unhelpful illness behaviour reinforced by poorly thought out and unexplained investigation and treatment. Patients will follow surprisingly little of your advice unless you really make an effort.

In general practice

People want to make sense of any perceived change in their health. You may be the first person to whom they tell that particular story, and it may not make much sense if it is squeezed into the 'medical model.'

People come to you for guidance, advice and treatment. Reasonable health promotion is OK, but be careful not to step over the line into overzealous lifestyle advice.

People are less informed than you think. Many procedures and screening programmes require much more sharing of understanding.

What doctors should know about communication

Oscar Wilde said of England and America that we were divided by a common language. The same could be said of doctors and patients. Most patients do not know the difference between a virus, a bacterium and an amoeba – they are all bugs. Most GPs use the virus versus bacteria issue to bolster their arguments about antibiotic prescribing. How many patients are using the same frame of reference? Peter Havelock, a GP friend, told me of the time he reviewed a recorded consultation with the patient, an elderly man. They watched it together, and at the end the old man made the following comments:

> Patient: Yes, Doc, I thought that were good, but I was just a bit unhappy about one thing. You said you were going to give me antibiotics and then at the end you didn't.
> Doctor: But I gave you penicillin.
> Patient: Oh, I didn't realise thems were antibiotics.

Patients have clear expectations of what will happen in conversations with doctors. A local radio show held a competition for the event you would most like to happen but which would be most unlikely to happen to you. One of the winners was 'going to your doctor with a sore throat and getting antibiotics without an argument about viruses.' The potential for misunderstandings between doctors and patients is unlimited.

Out of the mass of research work on communication with patients, the following stark truths emerge.

- The amount of explanation that a patient receives is directly related to their intelligence as perceived by the doctor.
- The lower the patient's social class, the less explanation is offered. Yet all patients from the highest to the lowest and the brightest to the more intellectually challenged want as much information as they can assimilate, and in a form that they can understand. This is a very big challenge to our profession.
- Patients' and doctors' perceptions of patients' problems differ from those expressed both before and after their consultations. Their perceptions about the consultation itself also differ.
- Asking questions only gets you answers. This is one of the problems with traditional history taking – a method of putting communication into a straitjacket in order to maximise pattern recognition.
- Doctors are likely to consistently overestimate their patients' understanding. Written information, pamphlets and leaflets are useful but poorly understood by the majority of the population. Other problems with written material include not being noticed, not being read and not being remembered.
- Doctors rarely talk to patients about the consequences of their illnesses. We do usually explain a little, but we rarely share what our patients think, and we also rarely check whether our patients understand. Sharing any type of management is still unusual. Our consultations are very one-sided.
- *To consult effectively you must search for your patient's agenda and reconcile this with your own agenda. This is a skilful process, and the outcome should be a shared understanding and a shared management plan.*

Let us now summarise again what you should seek to achieve in a consultation with a patient, in hospital or in general practice.

1 Discover the reason(s) why your patient has come to see you

To achieve this you will need to do the following.

- Try to understand your patient. To do this you will need to:
  - listen to them
  - obtain and use relevant social and occupational information
  - explore their health understanding
  - enquire about problems other than the presenting one.
- Try to understand the problem(s). To do this you will need to:
  - obtain additional information about critical symptoms and details of the medical history
  - assess your patient's condition by examination if appropriate
  - make a working diagnosis
  - assess the severity of the presenting problem.

2 Share understanding

To achieve this you will need to do the following.

- Share your findings with the patient.
- Tailor the explanation to the needs of the patient.
- Ensure that the explanation is understood and accepted by the patient.

3 Share decisions and responsibility

To achieve this you will need to do the following.

- Together with the patient, choose an appropriate form of management.
- Involve your patient in the management plan to the appropriate extent.
- Try to achieve a shared management plan.
- Ensure that the patient understands the plan.

4 Make effective use of the consultation

To achieve this you will need to do the following.

- Make efficient use of resources, including:
  - effective use of time
  - appropriate investigations
  - appropriate referral
  - appropriate concordant prescribing.
- Establish and maintain an effective relationship with your patient.
- Give opportunistic health advice where appropriate.
- Safety net effectively.

If you practise the completion of the above tasks, hone your present skills and learn some new ones as necessary, you will become a better doctor than you are now. Your patients should be happier and healthier, too. Good consulting.

Suggested reading

Since the early editions of this book were published, the concept of a reading list has been fundamentally changed by the Internet. Most articles now have electronically linked references, so there is no longer a need for a detailed list. What follows is a list of some of my favourite books and just a few modern review articles (from which further references can be obtained).

Essential

- Pendleton D, Schofield T, Tate P, Havelock P. *The Consultation: an approach to learning and teaching.* Oxford: Oxford University Press; 1984.
- Pendleton D, Schofield T, Tate P, Havelock P. *The New Consultation. Developing doctor–patient communication.* Oxford: Oxford University Press; 2003.
- Neighbour R. *The Inner Consultation.* 2nd ed. Oxford: Radcliffe Publishing; 2005.

Good value

- Helman C. *Suburban Shaman: Tales from Medicine's Front Line.* London: Hammersmith Press; 2006.
- Balint M. *The Doctor, his Patient and the Illness.* London: Tavistock Publications; 1957.
- Byrne P, Long B. *Doctors Talking to Patients.* London: RCGP Publications; 1976.

- Tuckett D, Boulton M, Olson C *et al. Meetings Between Experts.* London: Tavistock Publications; 1985.
- Pendleton D, Hasler J, editors. *Doctor–Patient Communication.* London: Academic Press; 1983.
- Ley P. *Communicating with Patients.* London: Croom Helm; 1988.
- Silverman J, Kurtz S, Draper J. *Skills for Communicating with Patients.* 2nd ed. Oxford: Radcliffe Publishing; 2004.
- Skrabanek P. *The Death of Humane Medicine.* London: The Social Affairs Unit; 1994.
- Drucquer M, Hutchinson S. *The Consultation Toolkit.* London: Reed Healthcare Publishing; 2000.
- Stewart M, Brown JB, Weston WW *et al. Patient-Centred Medicine: transforming the clinical method.* Oxford: Radcliffe Medical Press; 2003.
- Misselbrook D. *Thinking About Patients.* Newbury: Petroc Press; 2001.
- Edwards AGK, Elwyn G, editors. *Evidence-Based Patient Choice: inevitable or impossible?* Oxford: Oxford University Press; 2001.
- Downie R, Macnaughton J. *Clinical Judgement: evidence in practice.* Oxford: Oxford University Press; 2000.
- Salinsky J, Sackin P. *What Are You Feeling, Doctor? Identifying and avoiding defensive patterns in the consultation.* Oxford: Radcliffe Medical Press; 2000.

Three useful *British Medical Journal* issues

- Volume 7212. *Embracing Patient Partnership.*
- Volume 7417. *Communicating Risks: illusion or truth.*
- Volume 7419. *From Compliance to Concordance.*

A few recent articles on communication

- Little P, Everitt H, Williamson I *et al.* Observational study of effect of patient centredness and positive approach on outcomes of general practice consultations. *BMJ.* 2001; **322:** 908–11.

- Kidd J, Patel V, Peile E *et al.* Clinical and communication skills. *BMJ.* 2005; **330:** 374–5.
- Griffin SJ, Kinmonth A-L, Veltman MWM *et al.* Effect on health-related outcomes of interventions to alter the interaction between patients and practitioners: a systematic review of trials. *Ann Fam Med.* 2004; **2:** 595–608.
- Howie J, Heaney D, Maxwell M. Quality, core values and the general practice consultation: issues of definition, measurement and delivery. *Fam Pract.* 2004; **21:** 458–68.
- Stewart M. Reflections on the doctor–patient relationship: from evidence and experience. *Br J Gen Pract.* 2005; **55:** 793–801.
- Elwyn G, Edwards A, Hood K *et al.* and the Study Steering Group. Achieving involvement: process outcomes from a cluster randomized trial of shared decision-making skill development and use of risk communication aids in general practice. *Fam Pract.* 2004; **21:** 337–46.
- Roberts J. Describing the road to death. *BMJ.* 2005; **331:** E364–5.
- Kirk P, Kirk I, Kristjanson LJ. What do patients receiving palliative care for cancer and their families want to be told? A Canadian and Australian qualitative study. *BMJ.* 2004; **328:** 1343.

The ICE man cometh

In 1979, three Thames Valley Course organisers, Theo Schofield, Peter Havelock and myself, plus our new friend, social psychologist David Pendleton, first used the triumvirate of *ideas, concerns and expectations (ICE)* as the basis for understanding our patients' health beliefs, and started to include this concept in our day-release teaching. It led to the writing of the book *The Consultation: an approach to learning and teaching* (published by Oxford University Press in 1984). We have another version out now with a very similar message, *The New Consultation. Developing doctor–patient communication* (published by Oxford University Press in 2003). I have also written *The Doctor's Communication Handbook*. Over the years ICE has perhaps become an overused mnemonic, trotted out with little meaning by many hoping to please teachers and examiners. It is now time to redress the balance.

You see I am recovering from a severe attack of ideas, concerns and expectations. This relates to the fact that I have also been rather ill. Those of you who don't like illness stories will perhaps stop now, but let me try to persuade you to bear with me. My first idea was that I was too fat (17 stone). I was concerned about my nagging angina-like pain (previously but dubiously diagnosed as oesophagitis), and I expected that weight loss would make me feel better and perhaps improve the gout, too. Having tried every conventional diet in the books to no avail, this time the low-carbohydrate strategy seemed worth a try. It worked a treat. Within two weeks a youthful feeling returned, the gout went as did the 'angina', and a stone fell off. A life appeared ahead and the future beckoned. Ah hubris, always just around the corner. Unfortunately I have sick sinus syndrome and have been paced since 1977. Wires are fragile things with limited life spans and are difficult to remove. By the time of this saga I had four – three broken ones and a live one connected to the current box. One was 'tied off' below the skin in the upper right breast. This was no real problem as there was plenty of fat to cushion it (Mae West might have been envious), but as the fat evaporated the wire began to poke through the skin. What to do? There was a learned fear of cardiologists due to 25 years of interventions and different opinions. Then an idea – it's a breast problem, so get a nice plastic surgeon to snip the wire, easily done, a quick day case and no fuss. I was down to 14 stone now, more energetic than I had been for a decade, and the little grey cells were bubbling away with vigour now that they were freed from the custard of lethargy that had seemed to be engulfing them. But what are these night sweats and funny feelings in the chest? Over eight weeks of increasing lethargy and ineffective self-treatment the concern is clear – I know I have an infected wire, but I also know that to treat me properly they will have to take the whole lot out, and this is not an attractive prospect. Eventually my registrar makes the decision for me. She tells me that I will be dead if something is not done soon, and checks the c-reactive protein (CRP), which comes back at 219 mg/ml (normal range < 8 mg/ml). Paradoxically, this makes me feel better, as it proves I am not skiving. My ideas are that this will be a long job. My concerns are that I won't make it and my expectations are of an extremely unpleasant few weeks.

Let me say that from the cleaner to the consultant cardiologist everyone was kind beyond the call of duty, but implacable – all of them. They put an IV line in, warned me that I would need six weeks of treatment, and said that I probably had endocarditis and that first and foremost the old pacing system had to come out. Now as you know I write books on doctor–patient communication, so I tried some patient–doctor communication. 'What is it going to be like to take the old wires out?' 'Think of it as legalised GBH' said my fellow Geordie senior registrar with a smile. This honesty quieted me somewhat. 'Er, what about the risks?' 'Ah, only for old ladies, of course, there is tamponade, but the right ventricle is such a low-pressure system it's no real problem.' The insouciance of it all. There was no point in whinging.

'Er, the pain?' 'We'll give you what the Russkis gave the Chechens, that'll keep you quiet.' Well, it did, with added fentanyl a five-hour struggle felt like 45 minutes. Vaguely remembered feelings of tugging and the heart mildly objecting to being turned inside out were academic rather than emotional. However, I did get the feeling that all was not 100%.

'Well, how did it go?' I said brightly the next day to the assembled band at the foot of my bed. There was a brief but unmistakable dropping of eyelids, shuffling and forced smiles. 'Fine, just fine.' There was a strained attempt at humour. 'Shame your scrap value has collapsed.' And my friend the Geordie was detailed to come back with a slightly fuller version of the truth.

'We thought we might lose you, you know' was the opening gambit. 'I thought only old ladies died?' 'Well, yes, of tamponade, but it was the IVC (intravascular coagulation) that really worried us.' 'Eh?' 'Well, like toxic shock, all those wires with toxins on them being stripped off, too much and it all coagulates and that's it really.' My ideas on informed consent were shaken to the core. Was I pleased that I didn't know this risk beforehand? I decided that I was, and sank further into passivity. In the lull that followed the senior registrar filled the gap: 'Shame the wire snapped.' I felt like a stunned trout and let the fly dangle in front of me. 'You see there's a fragment we will need to take out.' 'Where?' was the best I could manage. 'Oh, it's just in the pulmonary artery, no real problem. We had better put you on fragmin (blood thinner) injections until we fish it out. The interventional radiologists are going to do it next week.' So that was all right then. My ideas about fragments of wire in pulmonary arteries were vague in the extreme, my concerns were also vague but much nastier, and my expectations of more pain and faffing about were 100% accurate. 'Fragment' turned out to be a euphemism for two and a half inches of something that looked like barbed wire, but was in fact a very frayed 25-year-old wire. I felt inexplicably better for having it removed.

'Is that it?' The eyelids drop again. My concernometer registers 'Oh shit' on a five-point scale. 'Well, there is another fragment . . . stuck in the right ventricle . . . would need open heart surgery . . . probably OK to leave it.' Now 'probably' is a word for doctors, it is not a good word for patients, but the repartee has dried up. The senior registrar fills the silence: 'Your creatinine is not too good, too much gentamycin so we will have to keep an eye on the renal failure first anyway.' Kidney failure and nasty fragments somewhere crucial? A Chagall-like vision of dead daffy-looking ducks floated by and the concernometer went off the scale, but no real sound came out other than a sort of John Mills *circa* 1945 propaganda film when his leg has just been blown off: 'Oh, that's a bit of a bugger, ah well . . .'. I am reminded of Kenneth Williams' famous rejoinder to the question 'Dammit man, where is your stiff upper lip?' 'Above this loose flabby chin.'

Weeks went by. I was allowed home to administer the IV antibiotics myself, much to the chagrin of the wonderful nurses, who were all firmly of the opinion that most doctors could not be trusted to wipe their noses let alone give complicated injections. I felt better, too – shame about the angina which had recurred on mild exertion, but spirits were up and I was not dead, the agonising gout had gone as the kidney function had improved, and the thought of going back to general practice, my patients and partners was an attractive one. Repeated echocardiograms showed no concretions, but the tricuspid valve was damaged, and my relative unfitness was ascribed to this. 'Get fit' was the message, so I did and within four weeks was walking the fells and the Roman Wall at Housteads for ten miles on a Saturday in January when the temperature was minus 5°C, with no angina to speak of. A check treadmill was arranged for the next week before going back to work, but that was just crossing the t's. I felt good, had no pacemaker for the first time in 25 years, and soon this would all be over and just a story. My concernometer had dropped to zero and my expectations were of a busy return to work. Did I mention hubris?

Even I could see that the ST segments were very wonky. The chest tightness was mild and I did do nine minutes, but the eyelids were down again. The consultant came and was solicitous and firm: 'Looks like stents . . . need angiography PDQ . . . in fact I have a cancellation – see you tomorrow.'

The ideas about stents are pretty good, or they could be worse, and the new antibiotic ones seem like a real step forward. The concerns that it might just be a little dodgy are not too bad, and the expectations of still getting back to work soon are OK. Another trip through the hospital on my back – I swear I could navigate this hospital just by looking at the ceilings. Much bonhomie followed by silence again. The television shows a picture I don't want to see. Why is there very little white dye getting down that big artery on the left ventricle? 'Peter, I am afraid you have a problem . . .' says a kind and slightly sad voice. Stenting is not possible, there is critical occlusion of the left main coronary artery, and the right system is not too good to boot. All that red wine to no avail. I was fairly fit half an hour ago, but now I am an invalid facing another major heart operation with all the uncertainties that that entails. He won't even let me go home because the narrowing is so critical, and bleating about walking the wall is just a waste of breath. 'Peter, which cardiac surgeon would you like?' Being a GP I know who I wouldn't like, coded responses pass between us, he smiles and says he would recommend the youngest who is a good communicator, with a further smile, almost a wink. This suits me fine, but being a patient I want him to be the best operator in the UK and I don't really care if he is ruder than Sir Launcelot Sprat. Ah, how values change.

So here I am writing this three weeks post quadruple coronary artery bypass graft and open heart surgery to remove the offending fragment, which was apparently not doing me any good, so the chest surgery could be construed as lucky in a perverse kind of way. I am afraid that my ideas, concerns and expectations are still a bit wobbly – they haven't settled from the operation yet. I think the expectations are the hardest things at the moment, but I will report back, God willing.

Peter Tate
Education for Primary Care 2003; **14**: 251–3.

Postscript, April 2006

I am now much improved, although retired from full-time general practice, taking the statin and watching the weight. Life is good.

spudtate@supanet.com

Index

Page numbers in *italic* refer to figures.